A WELL-DRESSED GENTLEMAN'S POCKET GUIDE

Oscar Lenius

PRION

First published in Germany by Lit Verlag, Munster
Published in Great Britain in revised form in 1998 by

Prion
an imprint of the
Carlton Publishing Group
20 Mortimer Street
London W1T 3JW

20 19 18 17 16 15 14 13 12 11

ISBN-13: 978-1-85375-569-9

Editor Richard Walker

Picture acknowledgements:
The Vintage Magazine Co. iv., viii., 66, 84, 98, 154, 164, 190

Printed in China

CONTENTS

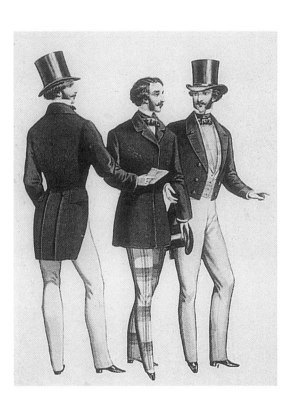

INTRODUCTION

THE GENTLEMAN'S ATTIRE is largely derived by descent from the hunting clothes of early 18th-century England. What we define as 'classic' style is a marriage of this tradition to the practical requirements of the present. It never has been static, but is an evolving accommodation.

The process can be said to have begun with Charles II, who in personally helping to define the suit in its early form was the first in a distinguished line of British royals to rule over matters sartorial. Subsequent arbiters were heirs to the throne, each in his turn a Prince of Wales. A century after Charles II, the prince destined to become George IV placed his seal upon the perfectionism of Beau Brummell. In the following century, the prince who would become Edward VII brought his trade to Savile Row, a small London street that under royal patronage became synonymous the world over with classical correctness in male dress.

Edward VII's handsome grandson, the uncrowned Edward VIII, rescued style from its starched Victorian strait-jacket by energetically promoting what he termed the 'dress soft' effect of soft-collared shirts and lounge suits, and bright, patterned tweeds and casual sweaters. His abdication on 11 December 1936 marked a sartorial watershed. Efforts to pass the mantle to his brother George VI failed, and the world moved on.

The male wardrobe is now big business affected by swirling global forces in an international market of designer labels. Yet these fashions are still anchored upon the founding precepts of Savile Row. And while the parvenu might dress to extremes in response to the dictates of fashion, the accomplished dresser can still cleave to that happy medium in line and cut which circumscribes the eternal verities of style.

Style is more than pure appearance. It is the conveyance of an aura of distinction, as hard to define as it is easy to recognize. Good tailoring is basic, of course, but then comes the hard question of choice.

The clothes of the gentleman must suit the occasion, must suit each other, and must suit the particular individual to the extent that they project his personality to advantage, while providing poise and a sense of confident well-being.

The rules which have grown out of tradition should guide rather than govern, and one should beware of creating too studied an effect. It is the well-dressed man who is noticed, never his clothes.

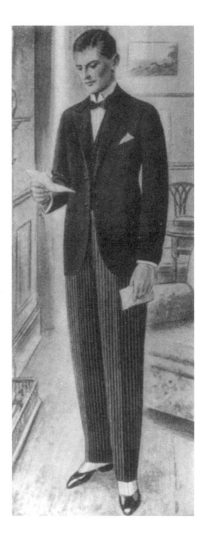

SUITS

HISTORY

The invention of the modern suit, as a matching set of clothes, is usually put down to the common sense of the English country gentleman of the late 18th century, acting in concert with his uniquely skilled London tailor. The story, however, goes much further back.

The word 'robe' once referred to a set of garments, and we know from the accounts of Edward III, father of the Black Prince and foe of France, that his 'Great Wardrobe' contained numerous 'suites of clothes'. A 'suite' then could consist of up to half-a-dozen garments. Reducing this to a practical and stylish three or two pieces was to be the work of more than 500 years.

It was in Edward III's reign that the notion of tailoring first took hold: the word itself did not come into use until very late in the 13th century. Prior to that, clothes were not shaped, through cutting and construction, but hung more or less loosely, so that everyone looked rather like a relative of Friar Tuck.

One of the earliest effects of the Italian Renaissance, when humanism replaced the other-worldly Middle Ages, was to change the way people wanted to look. The loose robe or tunic was short-ened, tightened, snipped and stitched to the con-tours of the body. There is a contemporary poetic description of Sir Gawain's Green Knight displaying 'his hips and haunches...elegantly small' in a tunic 'tight at the waist/At back and at breast his body was broad.' As exact a description of the sartorial ideal as would ever be written.

The New Look proved a popular sensation, to the discomfort of men in holy orders who were quick to equate tight clothing with loose morals. French commentators attributed the English victory at the Battle of Crecy in 1346 to divine retribution against their side for dressing so indecently.

Italy lost the style lead to Spain, which instituted the sombre elegance of black, which in England was combined with cream, still today a formula for for-mal grace. Spain in turn ceded cultural dominance to France, whose 'Sun King' Louis XIV presided over an age of extreme ostentation. From powered wig to silver-buckled shoes, the gentleman was a chrysalis encased in brocades and satins, velvet and lace.

This did not sit well with a reluctant guest of his. Charles II, upon returning from exile after the Cromwellian interlude, determined to break the English of a habit of slavishly aping the French. He wanted something that was distinctly English, and that would end the tyrannic vagaries of fashion by staying in style indefinitely.

Samuel Pepys, himself the son of a tailor, recorded in his diary some of the key moments. On 3 February 1661, Pepys stepped out for the first time in his 'coate', that being 'the manner now among gentlemen'. This coate was a knee-length adaptation of a loose riding garment that in its new form replaced the padded doublet, itself a development of the original tunic.

Step two, in 1666, was the introduction of the 'vest'. Straight-cut, close-fitting, it was promoted personally by the king, and soon everybody who was anybody was wearing vests, or waistcoats, as they came to be called. The third and final step was to replace bulging French 'petticoat breeches' with a much narrower style, cut to the knees. The result, by 1670, was a three-piece suit, first in a line extending to the present day.

The French were not about to capitulate. Regulation wear at the Court of Versailles was still the outfit required of high society. It was at this point that the English country gentleman made his great contribution to the future of civilisation.

Unlike their doomed French cousins, the upper classes of England were loath to waste time at Court, much preferring to romp about their country estates. Hunting was their particular pleasure, and since it was hardly possible to mount a horse in courtly garb, something had to give. Coat-skirts were cut away at the front, leaving only tails at the back.

Brocades and velvets were discarded for plain cloth cut for comfort and ease of movement. A hard-wearing woollen riding coat worn by country folk caught the aristocratic eye. Comparatively loose-fitting, and with a high, turned-down collar, it was adapted for the drawing-room. Colours sobered, to the extent that a shade of brown became so common in the 1770s that it entered the language as a description of anything dull or monotonous. That shade was 'drab'.

The mood was infectious. For his seminal novel of romance and tragedy, *The Sorrows of Young Werther*,

Goethe in 1774 dressed his protagonist in a blue English tailcoat. From such an auspicious endorsement, this 'Werther dress' would be gradually accepted in Germany and eventually become standard throughout Europe.

The scene was set for the most famous partnership in sartorial history. In 1795, an arrogant youth named George Bryan Brummell made the acquaintance of the Prince of Wales, the future George IV, and proceeded to mesmerise him with his wit and an extraordinarily fastidious sense of style. Though profligate and self-indulgent, the Prince as pupil proved the perfect conduit for the teachings of the immortal Beau Brummell, whose word on the exact cut of a coat or the starching of a stock could consequently not be denied.

Brummell set new rules to cope with new circumstances. A gentleman's appearance had previously depended upon the richness of the material upon his back: it mattered not that the clothes were often badly made and ill-fitting, and not always particularly clean. Quality now became something one knew when one saw it, but was difficult to describe. It came down to cut and fit, to exquisitely minute detail, and to the sometimes mystical relationship of a man with his tailor. It has been said of Brummell that his clothes seemed to melt into each other with the perfection of their cut and the quiet harmony of their colour. Without a single point of emphasis, everything was distinguished. And he preached an immaculate state of cleanliness.

Essential allies in all of this were the weavers of fine English cloth and the tailors of London, who developed techniques for moulding the cloth as a sculptural medium. Brummell's arrogance and cruel wit eventually alienated the Prince and gambling brought on his ruin, but his dictates endure as the essential code of the well-dressed gentleman to this day. Even his preference in colour – blue – would endure to the extent that the navy suit became the uniform of millions through much of the 20th century.

Through the 19th century the tailcoat evolved into formal dress. A looser 'frock coat' replaced the tailcoat as everyday wear, only in its turn to gradually give way to a still easier arrangement initially intended only to 'lounge' in. The suit as we know it had evolved.

MATERIAL

WOOL

Pure new wool is the stuff of the traditional, classic suit. People slung sheepskins over their backs before learning from around 3500 BC to spin and process the fleece. By the Middle Ages, England and Spain dominated the wool trade. Wool financed early Spanish exploration and it comprised 80 per cent of England's exports in Elizabethan times.

Wool is warm: it insulates, protecting against heat as well as cold. It is water-absorbent, soaking up perspiration and circulating it back into the environment, and it is also water-resistant thanks to a waxy fibre-coating. It is hard to set alight, and merely smoulders. It is durable and resilient. It responds well to a steam iron.

In general, the best wool is produced by merino sheep, a breed of Spanish-Moorish origin introduced to Australia at the end of the 18th century. Merino wool is fine and very wavy. Among hundreds of other breeds, long-wool sheep of English origin, such as Cotswolds, are often cross-bred with the short-fleeced merinos, while Scottish Cheviots make fine tweeds.

As well as class and quality of the wool, distinctions stem from the methods of processing. Woollen yarns are made from fibres that are carded (separated) and then tangled into a rough, loose mass, which is then twisted into yarn. Worsted yarns are made by combing the woollen fibres until they lie straight, then drawing and tightly twisting the smooth yarn; the name comes from the Norfolk village of Worstead.

Suit fabric may be made from worsted or woollen yarns, or both in combination, or the yarns may be blended with cotton or silk, or man-made fibres may be introduced for special reasons.

In the weaving process, the threads of yarn are interlaced at right angles to each other. All woven fabrics are derived from variations of three basic weaves, of which two dominate in garment cloth. The most simple and common is plain weave, an over-and-under pattern formed by the alternate interlacing of the warp (vertical) and weft (horizontal) yarns. Twill weave is created by interlacing the warp and weft so that the fabric has a diagonal slant.

FLANNEL

Famously supple, loosely woven cloth with a lightly-brushed surface. The name is probably of Welsh origin. There are both carded (woollen) and worsted flannels made of fine merino wool. Flannel should not be worn continuously over long periods, but allowed time to 'rest'. It also tends to peel under heavy friction, which is why it is advisable to have two pairs of trousers for every matching jacket. So-called chalk stripe fabrics are always of flannel, sometimes in a variety of blends with cotton and man-made fibres.

WORSTED SUITINGS

These are made in a range of weights, with a strong tendency towards ever lighter fabrics. Before the Second World War, the demand was for suitings of 17-20 ounces to the cloth yard. By the 1950s, the average was down to 14-16 ounces and the tendency has continued. Summer suitings may be of 8 ounces or less.

Fancy worsteds are known by the name given to the distinctive weave of each. They include:

HOUNDSTOOTH

This twill-weave effect is achieved by intertwining four dark threads with four light threads (commonly black and white) to create a small checkered pattern that might be said to resemble the teeth of a dog.

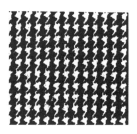

BARLEYCORN

The blurry little 'corn' triangles that characterise this twill-weave cloth, is achieved by contrasting the warp and the weft threads. As well as being appropriate for business and general day-wear suiting, barleycorn in lambswool or cashmere makes a pleasing sports jacket.

HERRINGBONE

Twill-weave with threads running alternately to left and right to form an inverted-V design that could be construed as the bones of a fish. This is a popular style for suits and sports jackets.

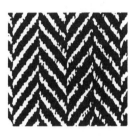

PINSTRIPE

This classic suit pattern is achieved by using white, grey or other contrasting yarns in series in a very fine worsted cloth. Anthracite, light grey, and middle to dark blue is the standard pinstripe range.

PICK-AND-PICK (SHARKSKIN)

Smooth, twill-weave worsted suiting with a dark-and-light 'salt-and-pepper' effect. A favourite with businessmen which has become available in lighter weights.

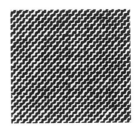

GLEN CHECK

Also known as Glenurquhart, this is one of the 'district checks', originally livery designs for 19th-century Scottish landowners. It was a favourite of Edward VIII when Prince of Wales. It is most often in black and white and is suitable for daytime and business suits.

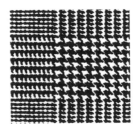

SAXONY

This milled twill from carded yarns is usually rendered as a Glencheck. It is more woolly and rough than a worsted and can be classified at the finest end of the tweed spectrum. The firm, closely-woven cloth often features a silk stripe and makes a smart suiting for town as well as country.

TWEED

The generic name for a very wide variety of stubbly coarse woollen cloths, typically of multicoloured carded yarns and twill construction. The name was born out of a clerical error. A scribbled invoice for some bolts of Scottish 'tweel' was misread as 'tweed', and so it has renamed, to be regularly mis-associated with the river of that name.

Tweel was a Scots rendering of twill, and the cloth so-named was a heavy homespun cloth that had been woven for centuries in Scotland and which was beginning to take the fancy of London gentry, who came upon it on their shooting and fishing trips up north. The royal association with Balmoral did the rest. Tweed clothing became tweeds, an important element of leisure wear.

Irish tweeds tend to be the more colourful, with large patterns, whereas Scottish tweed patterns tend towards the very small. The most famous tweed is Harris tweed, rugged as the island it came from, and still does if bearing the famous Orb Mark of the Harris Tweed Association. It is very bulky, for hard country wear. Shetland is much softer and finer; with a loose texture, it creates sports clothing of character, though less endurance.

CHEVIOT

Very hard wearing, grainy and yet with a lustre, this tweed type in a fishbone-patterned weave is one of the heavier of classic cloths. It was originally produced exclusively from wool of the Cheviot breed.

PLAID

Boxlike patterns with bright and dark checks produced by the cross-hatching of yarn-dyed fibres. In sufficiently sober checks, particularly in black and white, they make ideal suit patterns. Plaids also include Scottish tartans.

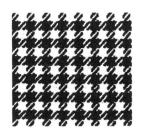

GABARDINE

A smooth, cloth in fine to medium worsted yarns that is so tightly woven it is soil-resistant and almost water-resistant. The twill rib is pronounced due to a weave with more warp threads than weft. It is usually in solid colours. This cloth is a popular suiting for all uses, including formal dress, but it is wise to check on the quality since this can vary.

TROPICAL

A plain-weave worsted made with high-twist two-play yarn . An airy suiting for summer wear and hot climates, light and yet sturdy and crease-resistant.

COTTON

Unless one subscribes to theories of a prehistoric global culture, cotton cultivation developed separately in the Middle East and South America very long ago. The name derives from the Arabic *qutn* and some cotton fabrics still bear the names of Asian cities with which they were identified.

Cotton is a tender plant requiring a moisture-retaining soil and 200 frost-free days, at the end of which the seed pod bursts open to reveal a tangled mass of fluffy fibres – raw cotton.

The Moors introduced cotton to Spain and returning Crusaders spread it further. East India Company imports of Oriental fabrics completed the job, but cotton production was necessarily limited until the invention in 1793 of the cotton gin, a machine that vastly reduced the labour of separating the seeds from the cotton 'boll'.

Cotton clothes are durable and practical: they absorb perspiration, do not irritate the skin, and can be washed repeatedly without damage. Cotton tolerates detergents and high temperatures – on the ironing-board, for instance – and it dyes easily. Against this, it creases and is not particularly warming. Treatments developed in the 19th century greatly improved its usefulness.

Cotton quality is determined by the length of the raw fibre, or staple. The best cottons come from southern Egypt and islands in the Caribbean region – the so-called Sea Island cotton, of which a variety known as Superfine St Vincent has fibres that can reach 50mm or more.

SEERSUCKER
This hot-weather suiting popular with Americans derives its name from a corruption of a Hindi phrase meaning 'milk and sugar' and was made with

silk when first discovered by the British in India. The puckered rough-smooth texture is attained by alternating the tension in the fibres.

VELVET
The name comes from vellus, Latin for fleece. Once exclusively made of silk, it is has a short, thick pile fabric. In plain or twill weave. it is used for jackets in the main.

CORDUROY
This familiar thick-ribbed fabric with a cut-pile surface is woven with sunken lines running lengthwise. The origin of the name, though often taken to be a corruption of French, is uncertain.

DENIM
This most American of fabrics is nothing of the kind. The name is a corruption of Nimes, the French city where it was first made and where it was termed 'Coton de Nimes', hence cotton denims. The word 'jeans' is a corruption of Genoese, Italian sailors from the port of Genoa being first to wear the type. The effect is achieved with a twill weave combining uncoloured weft threads with warp threads dyed indigo blue.

POPLIN

Heavier versions of this familiar fabric are used for jackets and trousers.

LINEN

The stalk of a particular variety of the flax plant is soaked and then 'scrunched' to extract the fibres. This used to be done by women beating the flax on the floor of their homes. They would then spin and weave the fibres and bleach the material by leaving it on a dew-covered lawn. All this has been long since automated.

Linen varies according to its origin. Irish linen is light and soft. Italian linens range from reddish to yellow-brown to gold, according to region. Belgian linen is shiny, and so on.

The crisp, grainy textured canvas (plain) weave of the nubbly thread is unique to linen, while its cooling effect in hot weather makes it ideal for summer wear. It has a notorious tendency to crease, but many value this as a 'natural' look.

IRISH LINEN

Long, regular fibres facilitate the weaving of a compact fabric highly valued for summer suits in solid colours. It does not crease as much as other linens.

ITALIAN LINEN

This is softer than Irish linen and the weave less uniform, thus suits in this material tend to have more 'character', though they will crease more easily.

There is also a linen gabardine in a type of twill weave that creates a non-traditional fabric which is slightly heavier and softer. Linen jackets may be made in so-called fancy linen, which is woven to achieve a very grainy effect somewhat akin to shantung silk. Indeed, it is often blended with silk or other fibre.

SILK

Silk is a very fine and shiny protein filament extruded by the mulberry-munching caterpillar of a moth, Bombyx mori, in the course of spinning its cocoon. Chinese tradition credits Hsi-ling-shi, teenage bride of the Emperor Huang Ti, with discovering the secret of the cocoon around 4700 years ago.

China kept that secret to itself for thousands of years, and finished silks transported along the fabled Silk Road created the first cultural ties between the Orient and the West. Two merchants disguised as monks managed to smuggle mulberry seeds and cocoons from China to Byzantium in 550AD and with the advance of Islam the secret reached Spain and then the rest of Europe in the Middle Ages.

Labour-intensive sericulture is still centred on China, which produces most of the world's raw silk. The cocoons are boiled and the filament extracted by an intricate reeling process, drawing upon the contents of several cocoons at once to form a continuous thread which is twisted, washed, and wound on a skein. Silk fabrics vary according to the thickness of the thread, the degree of twist and the type of weave.

Cool in summer, warm in winter, silk has a superior air about it that is most appropriate for festive evening wear and dinner jackets.

SATIN
First known as Zaitan, from a Chinese port of origin, this delicate silk fabric which is dull on one side and glossy on the other has lost some of its popularity and is now largely limited to waistcoats and the lining and trimming on formal evening wear.

SHANTUNG
This plain-weave, knotty fabric from coarse yarns is stronger than other silks and does not crease. With laundering, it becomes softer. It is used for dressy summer-weight suits and distinguished jackets. Beware inferior shantungs made from silk waste. A silk and wool twill creates a durable suit or jacket fabric. Silk plain-weave produces a lighter and glossy summer jacket. If closely woven, it may be referred to as silk poplin.

PRECIOUS FIBRES
The cashmere suit and the vicuna jacket need no descriptive phrases — the names have become synonymous with comfort and luxury.

Some have been precious since antiquity. Mohair was used to weave the curtains of the Temple tabernacle in Biblical times, cashmere shawls were prized by the Mongols, and Inca priests wore vicuna cloaks. In the Western world, the English gentleman was first to find superior merit in cashmere (Beau Brummell's tastes ran to white cashmere waistcoats) and camel-hair.

This was observed by richer Americans, who from the 1930s strove to emulate and then to out-dazzle in materials for which they were prepared to pay any price.

Most of these fabrics are made from the soft under-coat of creatures equipped to endure harsh climates. In some cases the natural colours are so attractive that they are rarely dyed.

CASHMERE

Worsted cashmere woven from the choicest under-coat of an Asian mountain goat is very light and yet almost as hardy as wool and not subject to the 'pilling' (furring) often associated with cashmere. Carded cashmere is very soft, but less secure. Cashmere is commonly blended with other materials for daytime and business suits.

MOHAIR

This fabric noted for its sheen comes from the hair of the Angora goat, a breed that originated in Turkey. Its elegant drape and crisp feel recommend it for business as well as formal wear. Mohair is also woven with a worsted wool to create a lustrous and durable summer suiting.

BABY ALPACA

The first shearing of this Andean member of the camel family produces a soft, silky fibre of distinctive quality. Apart from its rich lustre, fabric woven from this material is supple and light as a feather, yet surprisingly robust.

VICUNA

This famously expensive, soft and warm material comes at a price – the small, elusive vicuna, a close cousin of the alpaca, is killed for its fleece. Vicuna fabric is normally in a twill weave. It is not to be confused with a merino wool fabric woven to simulate vicuna and called by that name when made into morning coats and other garments.

FIT

Fit is the top priority in the acquisition of a suit. An ill-fitting suit is a miserable object, no matter how sumptuous the cloth or correct the style. Only, it is more complicated than that. Perfect fit is not the point – indeed, it would be in most cases a profound embarrassment. Rather, the object is to sculpt upon one's less-than-perfect torso a set of raiment that aspires to a particular ideal.

Tailors do not talk of style and fit, but of 'line' and of 'balance', which means the hang of the jacket and the way it moves – effortlessly – with the wearer. These are the qualities that distinguish the craft-tailored suit and which for generations have drawn men of distinction and discernment to Savile Row.

Matters have been muddied of late by great advances in industrial suit manufacture, aided in part by computer technology, and by the proliferation of high-profile 'designer' labels. One should bear in mind that in buying a designer suit, one is buying a style and a taste – a name – that may or may not be appropriate, while possibly paying as much or more than it would cost to have a suit hand-crafted for oneself alone.

With a bespoke suit, the choice of material is unlimited and one can indulge personal whims in styling and detail, under the close supervision of an expert cutter able to make the best out of the circumstances of one's particular build. Physical defects can be whittled away by clever tailoring, and attributes emphasised. Finally, a bespoke suit is built to last. Some of the Duke of Windsor's suits were hand-me-downs from his father, George V, and are estimated to have lasted 60 years.

Against this, it takes commitment and time and is in a sense more of a gamble that purchasing something tangible, off the rack. One is dealing here with a person and not a machine. There can be a conflict of minds, leading to disappointment, and seeking out the right tailor is quite as onerous as picking the right solicitor or doctor.

Savile Row has been the arbiter of male elegance for the better part of 200 years, its influence reaching out to the entire world (indeed, the Japanese word for suit is *sebiro*), but not in isolation. Of several contesting styles, the American and the Italian are most prominent. The difference in each case lies in the shape of the shoulders, for upon this everything, literally, hangs.

Savile Row shoulders are soft and not particularly large, with little padding, and jackets have a distinct waist. A characteristic is the 'blade', a clever fullness at the shoulder blades perfected by Scholte, a Savile Row colossus of the early 20th century, allowing greater movement while contributing to a flattering Y-shape silhouette.

The American style is based on the sloping 'natural' shoulder and is epitomised by the straight-drop 'sack' look worn by New York and Boston nabobs for half a century. Italian style has tended towards extremes, such as short, tight jackets, but since the 1970s it has become hugely influential due in the main to the drive and influence of designer Giorgio Armani, whose so-called deconstructed style with lighter fabrics and less padding and meticulous tailoring influenced a move to a looser, softer line.

Within the compass of the two or three-piece, single or double-breasted classic suit, the wearer has considerable latitude of choice in such matters as pockets and vents and trouser dynamics. 'Double-breasted' signifies an overlap of fabric in the jacket front, as against the simple fit-to-the-buttonline single-breasted jacket. It is much more subject to stylistic exploration than the more common single-breasted.

Flap pockets are appropriate for business suits and are combined with a breast welt pocket. Patch pockets are more sporty; patch pockets with box pleats are the most casual. The width of the lapel is a frequent victim of fashion's whim. A range of six to twelve centimetres will always stay 'correct'.

Town suits are traditionally in worsteds or flannel, country suits and sports jackets in tweed or flannel, but there has never been such choice in cloths, cottons and linen, and in blends that intrigue. The move to lighter construction was accompanied by the development in Italy of very light worsted Super 100s, while new weaving techniques have made possible lighter tweeds and a comeback of the tweed suit.

Black and white evening wear flatters all men because of the effect of its dramatic contrast, and the rule holds with colours in general. Gentlemen should shy away from shades that approximate their own colouring and look for the greatest possible contrast to their complexion. Greens and blues are generally most flattering to Caucasian skins and most certainly to the fresh-complexioned. A pale complexion is best set off against dark suiting.

Dark and thinly striped materials will help to 'slim-down' a portly figure, while thick stripes have the opposite effect. Light, or checked material gives 'bulk' to a thin person. Short gentlemen 'gain' height by having the waist of the jacket tailored high, or by having the pockets raised; placing the pockets lower than normal has the opposite effect. Wide lapels suit taller men. Narrow lapels appear to broaden a narrow chest. The tricks of the trade are endless. A good tailor knows them all.

CONSTRUCTION

Having a suit made for oneself is an experience like no other, especially if one patronises a Savile Row establishment. The air of dusty refinement, the long tables groaning with bolts of cloth and the swatch books crammed with cloth samples may daunt the neophyte, but he can rest assured that his business is mightily appreciated.

The fitting can take the best part of an hour, in a three-way-mirrored cubicle, an anatomical accounting attended by a fitter (or fitters) under the vigilant eye of the cutter, who is master of all Savile Row ceremony. Nothing dare be taken for granted; arms, for instance, are not necessarily of the same length. All the taped measurements are entered into a leather-bound ledger, there to remain for ever.

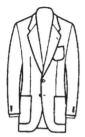 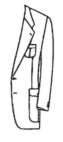 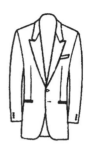

sports suits, three patch pockets, two patch pockets and breast welt pocket also possible	single-breasted two buttons, notched lapels, patch pockets with welted pockets	semiformal suit single breasted peaked lapels, box pleats

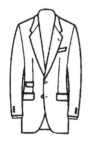 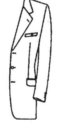 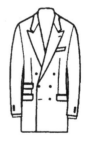

city and business suits single breasted, two buttons, notched lapels	single-breasted three buttons, notched lapels, flap pockets	double-breasted peaked lapels with or without ticket pocket

A paper pattern is constructed by the tailor and the cloth is marked with chalk according to the pattern, then it is cut (the correct word is 'struck') by the cutter. The struck sections are next passed to the tailors, usually one to a garment, who loosely baste them together with white thread. It is time for the first 'try-on', when corrections are made before the process moves to the 'forward' stage in which the suit is sewn into permanent shape.

The quality factory suit takes shape under radically different circumstances. Some manufacturers have computerised to a high degree. Video 'models' replace the craftsman's paper pattern and a computer-controlled machine cuts the cloth. From its computer data bank, the manufacturer can offer clients 'custom-made' garments to any style desired and faster than a traditional tailor can blink.

Whatever the provenance, inserting the canvases, tapes and paddings of the interlinings and finally the lining of a quality suit is a delicate, exacting procedure; ensuring no adverse reaction between the suit cloth and the interlinings is in itself complicated.

The hand-sewn canvas is made of a mix of natural fibres, including goat hair and hemp, layered at the shoulders and completed with strips of haircloth, which is made of cotton and horse-hair. A small pad is added to lend shape to the shoulders and help define the shoulder-line. Light cotton tapes are placed at critical points to help in the forming of the garment and in the curving of collar and arm-holes. The lining itself is not made of silk as it once was, but usually of a light artificial fabric, the most highly esteemed being a special bright, resistant type of filament, Rayon.

As a general rule, the more hand sewing, the superior the suit. Hand sewing the lapels to the underlining in the interest of achieving a perfect 'roll', and hand-stitched jacket borders, are signs of quality. Pressing is a critical, step-by-step process throughout the jacket's creation. All ironing is by hand in a tailor's shop, whereas machines give shape to a factory suit, with only the final finishing by hand.

Little or no mention has been made of the trousers, since they are so much simpler to make than the jacket that the work is often contracted out by leading bespoke tailors, although this is rarely mentioned to clients.

TESTING THE BOUQUET

A fine suit is somewhat like a fine wine, whose bouquet can only be fully appreciated by the connoisseur, but it behoves a gentleman to make himself aware of what to look for and what to require, especially if he is spending a substantial sum on a factory product, no matter how famous the label.

A quick tip is to check the buttons, which should be made from horn, not plastic, and in the case of a high-quality garment those on the sleeve should have functioning button-holes. Another indicator is the thickness of the seams: the greater the thickness, the poorer the quality. The lining needs to be closely examined; in the case of cheaper suits it was applied at the start and the jacket in effect built upon it. Still another indicator is the presence of tapes, evidence of careful construction.

The most drastic difference in quality is often difficult for the client to immediately discern, although it can show in a curious stiffness around the chest, lapels and some other areas. In a process known as 'fusing', some factory-made suits are glued together with thermo-adhesives in place of traditional interlinings. The initial effect might be excellent, but over time the glue dries out and the fabric starts to 'bubble' like blistered paint.

FORMAL WEAR

HISTORY

The tailcoat, 'tails', is the most formal of all garments, the required uniform of the grand ball. In the code of the formal invitation, it is what is implied by the imperious instruction: 'white tie'.

This is what has become of the original coat snipped into shape for easier riding by 18th-century country squires. It has changed little. It achieved great popularity in the first decades of the 19th century as an all-purpose 'dress coat'. By the 1860s it was strictly evening dress.

STYLE

The tailcoat is double-breasted, though never buttoned, remaining open on a low-cut white waistcoat made of stiff honeycomb cotton (pique), just visible beneath the jacket, and a stiff wing-collar shirt with starched, studded front, and white pique bow tie.

The black-and-white starkness provides the perfect foil for the colours of the ladies' gowns. Midnight blue, which appears intensely black under artificial light, is the only alternative option. In tying the bow (no easy task because of the starch), hands need to be immaculately clean to avoid leaving marks. The arrangement is directly descended from Beau Brummell's starched cravats, which may lend some consolation to one's labours.

Once everything is in place, an important consideration is management of one's tails, which are never to be sat upon, but carefully placed over the side or back of the chair.

Tails are also the work clothes of waiters (who wear black bows, be it noted, lest one commit a monumental social gaffe) and of musicians. When marvelling at the freedom of movement afforded the symphonic conductor, one should be aware that his armhole is specially cut with this in mind.

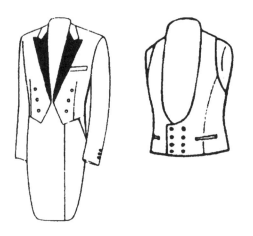

DINNER SUIT

HISTORY

One state removed from 'white tie' splendour, the 'black tie' dinner suit is the workhorse of formality, the only element of dress wear that the gentleman of average means is likely to own rather than hire.

The dinner jacket – the d.j. – is known to the French, Germans and Italians as the smoking jacket. Both names reflect its early uses. To the Americans, it is the Tuxedo, and therein lies a bone of contention.

In the 1880s, an evening version of the lounge suit, the 'dress lounge', was introduced. Usually it was made of the same black material as the tailcoat, and the jacket had a roll collar with satin-faced lapel. It answered the Victorian gentleman's desire to ease back on formality when at his club, say, or when passing the port and puffing a cigar on country-house weekends – whenever, that is, ladies were not present.

The problem lies in determining how and when the dress lounge became the dinner suit. In England, credit goes to the Prince of Wales, the future Edward VII, for donning one in Monte Carlo when he grew weary of sitting at the gaming tables in stiff starch.

In the United States, the honour is accorded tobacco tycoon Griswold Lorillard, who on 10 October 1886 dared to attend the Autumn Ball of the élite Tuxedo Park Club outside New York in a short black jacket instead of the requisite tails. The shock-horror gave way to emulation as fellow members ordered similar jackets from their tailors. Tuxedo became a new word in Websters Dictionary.

Deep in the ledgers of Henry Poole, the Savile Row tailors, there is an entry to the effect that just such a garment as Griswold wore was made for the Prince of Wales in the previous year, 1885, but wait - the origin of the dinner jacket has also been linked with the Homburg jacket, from Germany. The jury is out on the issue, and probably will remain so.

By 1900, in England, the dress lounge was being worn with a black bow tie, while in the U.S. the tuxedo was the subject of experimentation in various styles and materials, including already a white 'Tux'. All of this activity combined in the emergence of the dinner jacket-cum-tuxedo as the thing to wear at dinner parties and the theatre. Whatever the role of Edward VII, it was his grandson, the next Prince of Wales, who really established its popularity.

STYLE

The blacker-than-black magic of very dark blue under electric light was discovered by the Prince and his 1920s set. By comparison, plain black appears drear and dead. The disadvantage is that midnight blue cannot take daylight, so either one must maintain two outfits, or be content to lead the social life of a Count Dracula.

The dinner suit offers scope for individuality within the context of formality. The knack is in going so far, but no further. Hardy Amies, couturier and sartorial gadfly, believes for instance in sporting a coloured handkerchief, arguing that 'to show a white handkerchief is to show a white flag in the battle of life.' Surely the soundest advice comes from a 1960s manual published by the *Tailor and Cutter*: "If a coloured bow or a coloured waistcoat is introduced, great care must be taken they add some distinction to the outfit other than drawing comment and attention to the wearer."

A waistcoat is optional with the dinner jacket, and there is the jaunty alternative of the cummerbund, the waist sash first adopted by army officers serving in India. Cummerbunds are most flattering to the tall or slim. The portly are advised that black is not only traditional but has a slimming effect.

White dinner jackets for hot weather can be worn with a shawl collar and may be slightly longer and easier fitting than the black jacket. It is for open air social gatherings, e.g. at garden parties during the summer, or on sea voyages.

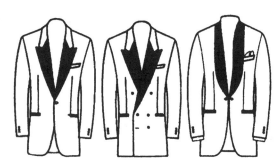

MORNING SUIT

HISTORY

The morning coat, the tailcoat of daytime, made its appearance in the 1890s, adapted from a much earlier design and promoted as a dressy, yet less formal alternative to the frock coat. Already it had its distinctive curved-back 'skirt', initially with three to four buttons instead of just one. This was strictly business attire. It gradually assumed its present duties after the frock coat died out with the Great War.

STYLE

In its original role, the morning suit took two forms – a black coat with striped or checked trousers and contrasting waistcoat, or a fully matching three-piece suit. It still takes two forms – black, with striped trousers and grey waistcoat, or completely light grey. The all-grey effect, top hat included, was once an exclusive feature of the Royal Enclosure at Ascot and Derby Day at Epsom. Now it lends distinction to many a summer wedding, though it must be said that gentlemen generally look better in black and that the all-grey suit is unknown on the Continent.

Americans and Germans call the morning coat a

'cutaway.' To the Italians, it is a 'tight', a term with which some unfortunates may concur. Since morning suits are generally hired these days, the priority must be to ensure that jacket and waistcoat allow breathing room and still have a balanced fit.

WAISTCOAT

HISTORY

This is the only garment to have been created by royal proclamation, and thus the only garment whose origin can be precisely dated. The date is Sunday October 7 1666. We know so because that assiduous civil servant Samuel Pepys entered it in his diary: 'The King hath yesterday in Council declared his resolution of setting a fashion for clothes, which he will never alter. It will be a vest, I know not well how.'

Pepys went to Westminster Hall the following Monday to find out. Charles II modelled the new style in person. This very first vest (a name still used by tailors, and Americans) was 'of black cloth and pinked with white silk under it.' Sober and comparatively simple, it flew in defiance of the extravagant dictates of Versailles and was thus part of a calculated strategy to undermine French influence.

The idea was not original, but based upon 'the Persian mode', a fad for the exotic brought back by English visitors to the Court of Shah Abbas. The Persian vest as adopted by the Court of St James was sleeved and long - longer, even, than the coat worn over it, but gradually it became shorter, to just above the knee, to mid-thigh, to the top of the thigh, and finally, by 1790, to the waistline, where it has remained ever since. It was sleeveless from the 1750s and in all but minor detail (such as the provision of a watch-chain hole, circa 1880) had become the waistcoat as we know it.

Despite the frugal intentions of its royal sponsor, in the course of the 18th century the waistcoat became an excuse for gorgeous display, with up to 20 buttons on parade. Beau Brummell, ever the purist, advocated pure white in waistcoats, but his was a lone voice. George IV owned around 300, and tucked his ever-increasing girth into ever more sumptuous creations.

Even in the grip of Victorian sobriety, the fancy waistcoat endured as an outlet for individual creativity. A gentleman's wardrobe properly contained upwards of a dozen in a self-indulgent riot of spots, stripes and floral patterns rendered in all manner of material and audacious colour.

The circumstances of the 20th century were to conspire against the waistcoat. Advances in home insulation, central heating and the 'saloon' car encouraged a shedding of superfluous clothing, while the emergence of the highly adaptable sweater, plus wartime austerity and clothes rationing combined to all but deal a death blow.

All, but…from the 1960s it began a slow recovery in both its incarnations, as raison d'etre of the three-piece suit and as a casual accessory. One factor has been the comeback of the single-breasted suit with trousers cut high to receive braces, for the belted, low-slung mode made it all but impossible to wear a waistcoat without ugly folds of shirt extruding.

STYLE

The classic six-button, single-breasted waistcoat with four pockets is suitable for any occasion. It has an adjustable back-strap to facilitate loosening and tightening. The back is made of the same material as the suit lining, or else it is of satin.

There is a custom which requires one to leave the bottom button undone. This is said to be because Edward VII (died 1910) left his bottom button undone. The king's grandson maintained that it came about by chance, when one day he forgot to do up the last button and his subjects mistook it for a style indicator. Others would have us believe that it was a function of the king becoming corpulent, but the fact of the matter is that for some reason undone waistcoat buttons have been in vogue since the 18th century, at least. It is more comfortable with the first button undone, giving the body more room and avoiding stretching the cloth.

The waistcoat has survived because it adds gravitas to the single-breasted suit, because it offers one an opportunity to cut a dash and make a statement, because it holds the tie in place and keeps the shirt neat and tidy, because it lends an efficient appearance to working in shirt-sleeves, because it is a neat place to store small change and pens, not to mention being the only place for a watch and chain...

Every gentleman in a 'weskit' has reasons of his own. The eminent Victorian, Edward Bulwer-Lytton summed matters up with ponderous exactitude. The waistcoat, he observed, "though apparently the least observable (garment) influences the whole appearance more than anyone not profoundly versed in the habilatory arts would suppose".

To avoid habilatory opportunity turning to tragedy, one must beware certain pitfalls:

Only a small segment of waistcoat, revealing no more than the top button, should under normal circumstances be visible above the jacket. Any greater exposure detracts from the tie and can cause discord sufficient to ruin the effect of the entire ensemble. Down below, if one is wearing a trouser-belt, it is essential that the waistcoat entirely cover the belt. Beware, above all, of a gap developing between waistcoat and trousers.

Waistcoats, high-point of the tailor's craft, are nowadays available off-the-peg in all manner of fabrics and designs. It is safest to wear these with other separates, but be fastidious in selecting a garment with no hint of that looseness at the waist or bagging at the front that would make its lack of pedigree obvious.

That said, it is remarkable the transformation that can be wrought upon the most ordinary of informal two-piece suits by the addition of just the 'right' unmatching waistcoat, so judicious experimentation is recommended.

CONSTRUCTION

While similar in form and tailoring to the suit jacket, the waistcoat is technically the most challenging garment, and the most difficult garment to construct satisfactorily.

It is required to lie flat as a pancake on a circumference as contoured as a potato, maintaining a 'touch-fit' that is nowhere tight. Since this is also the most discretionary of acquisitions – the one most subject to swings in popularity – it is small wonder that the specialist vestmaker is a rare and valued creature.

Style	Buttons	Lapel	Pockets
Tailcoat	double-breasted unbottoned	faced with satin peaked lapels	only breast welt pocket
Dinner jacket	single-breasted	peaked or shawl collar	welted pockets
	double-breasted	peaked	breast welt pocket
White Dinner jacket	single-breasted	peaked or shawl collar	welted pockets
	double-breasted	peaked	breast welt poc
Cutaway	single-breasted	peaked, 1 button fastening	only breast welt pocket
Semiformal suit	single-breasted	notched or peaked	flap pockets or welt pockets
	double-breasted	peaked	breast welt pockets
City or business suit	single-breasted	notched or peaked	flap pockets
	double-breasted	peaked	breast welt poc
Sports suit	single-breasted	notched	patch pocket norfolk pocket or welted pockets with breast welt pocket

	Colour	Pattern	Material	Trousers
ith e vent	black midnight blue	self-coloured	mohair/ wool	without turn-ups double silk braids
	black midnight blue	self-coloured	mohair/wool/ silk	without turn-ups single silk braids
	white écru	self-coloured	mohair/wool/ silk	without turn-ups double silk braids
ength	anthracite black	self-coloured marengo	wool	without turn-ups
vents hout ents	dark grey dark blue black	self-coloured stripes fil-à-fil	wool/ mohair/ flannel/ tropical	with or without turn-ups, double-beasted always with turn-ups
r ents	grey blue brown	glen check striped houndstooth fil-à-fil plaid herringbone	wool/ lambswool/ cotton/ linen/ flannel/ tropical/ gabardine/ cashmere/ Cheviot	with turn-ups
r centre	brown olive beige	glen check houndstooth plaid mousetooth herringbone	wool/ cashmere/ cotton/ linen/ shetland/ cheviot/ tweed/ lambswool	with turn-ups

Style chart	Suit
Semiformal occasions (opening days, opening of a shop)	dark, double-breasted, or single-breasted with waistcoat, flap pockets, trousers without turn-ups, double-breasted always with turn-ups
Formal occasions (small fesivities, receptions during the day and in the evening)	black, double-breasted or single-breasted with waistcoat, flap pockets, trousers without turn-ups, double-breasted always with turn-ups
Festive occasions during the day (weddings, funerals, receptions)	morning suit, black or marengo, single-breasted with waiscoat, flap pockets, morning suit-trousers without turn-ups
Festive indoor occasions in the evening (ballet, theatre, dinner)	dinner jacket, black, midnight blue, single-breasted or double-breasted with shawl collar or peaked laples, trousers without turn-ups with silk braids
Festive occasions in the open air in the evening (summer party, sea voyage)	dinner jacket, white or écru single-breasted or double-breasted peaked lapels or shawl collar, welted pockets, dinner jacket trousers
Very formal occasions during the day (weddings, funerals, receptions)	morning suit black, or marengo, peaked lapels, one-button fastening, knee-length tails, trousers without turn-ups in grey, or striped grey waistcoat, black for mourning
Very formal occasions in the evening (gala, dinner, state receptions)	tail-coat, peaked lapels faced with silk, tails with middle vents, trousers with double silk braids without turn-ups

t	Tie
e, French cuffs, lar collar	dark ground, discreet pattern, silk rep, crêpe de Chine
e, French cuffs, lar collar	pearl grey, self-coloured or finely patterned, black for mourning
e, French cuffs, lar collar	pearl grey, discreet pattern, black, white and grey, black for mourning
e, light blue, écru, ch cuffs, wing collar egular collar, front and concealed ket	hand-tied bow tie, black, blue, patterned, silk
er jacket shirt hite, light blue cru	black dinner jacket bow tie, silk
e with regular collar and ch cuffs or barrel cuffs	pearl grey or grey, black and white, plastron to coordinate with the wing collar
oat shirt with pleated front or piqué front, g collar, cuffs with onholes	white piqué bow tie, with wing collar, black for mourning

JACKETS AND BLAZERS

HISTORY

The name, jacket, derives from jaquet, a 15th-century borrowing from French, but the familiar pocketed jacket is a comparatively recent development.

True, Jane Austin found a 'shooting jacket' to be the most becoming of 'manly dresses' early in the century, but it was only from the mid-1800s that the jacket, as distinct from the frock coat or dress coat, began to come into its own. It was shorter than the coat and it had exposed pockets. It was cut to an easier, looser fit, and might be made of tweed or other novel fabric.

As the 'lounge jacket' with matching trousers evolved into the lounge suit, other jacket types proliferated. Two which were to endure were the pleated Norfolk jacket and the reefer, or yachting jacket.

The Norfolk jacket, which may have been cut first for the guests at one of the Duke of Norfolk's hunting parties, combined a relaxed fit with a smart appearance and was immensely popular through the first decades of the 20th century, usually in tones of reddish-brown. The double-breasted yachting jacket harked back to a short blue naval jacket named after a reefer, or midshipman. It also harked forward to the blazer.

There is a rollicking tale concerning the captain of an HMS *Blazer* fitting out his crew in dark blue serge jackets with brass buttons for Queen Victoria's coronation in 1837 – ergo, the blazer. Though the story often appears in sartorial manuals, it has no basis in fact.

Serge or flannel 'sports' jackets with patch pockets were being worn by cricket clubs and other sporting groups from the 1880s and it became a custom to decorate these with stripes in the club colours. Blazing bright, some of them were, and so they became known as blazers. The particular jacket which caused the coining of the word is said to have been in the vibrant colours of the Lady Margaret Boat Club in Cambridge.

Blazers with flannel trousers and straw boaters became an Edwardian symbol, joined subsequently by versions in navy blue with club badge on the breast pocket. From the 1920s, the blue blazer and flannels became an informal classic, just like the tweed jacket.

After the Second World War separates — sports jackets and odd trousers, augmented upon occasion by orphaned suit jackets — were increasingly worn in place of suits.

STYLE

The navy blazer and the tweed jacket loom large in virtually every gentleman's wardrobe, as they surely will for the foreseeable future. Indeed, some would regard the classic blazer as their single most essential item of apparel.

One must, however, place stress on that word 'classic'. There are constant, ill-advised attempts to toy with blazer design, as there are constant adaptations of the blazer shape to dubious purpose. These are to be shunned. The glory of the navy blazer rests with its purity of cut and cloth.

The classic double-breasted blazer has six buttons, side vents, side pockets and a breast pocket, and peaked lapels with a buttonhole in each. The buttons are metal: brass, gold, or silver. The effect is as dashing as it is correct. The single-breasted version, with either two or three buttons, is correct enough and is a most serviceable garment in itself, but it lacks the presence of its celebrated sibling.

The buttons should be plain, or very simply decorated, and the breast pocket must be bare. Badges only on a breast patch pocket, never as pure decoration, only in case of membership. As to fabric, a lightweight pure wool is correct, but there are a variety of options. A closely woven worsted with a slightly raised nap, flannel, or wool serge are all appropriate. Cashmere, too soft for trouser wear, is a further resplendent possibility.

If the navy blazer is essential, then the tweed jacket is the most loyal of garments, ever reliable and immensely useful in partnership with a trusty pair of flannel trousers.

The longevity of tweed is the stuff of legend, and clothing lore abounds with tales of tweed garments handed down the generations, and yet it is subject to abrasion and over time will fray at cuff and elbow. In consequence of this one weakness, the application of leather patches over the elbows is as appropriate as it is traditional, yet to incorporate patches when none is required, as with a new garment, is a 'design' conceit that must be frowned upon.

Tweeds are no longer the hairy brown monsters they once so often were. Nowadays they come in a broad range of subtle mixtures, of lovely lovats, flattering, soft blues and greens, and there are lighter weaves. The mix-and-match rules of casual separates are as obvious as they are simple to remember and the results will be rewarding. Wear a dark jacket with light trousers, and dark trousers with a light jacket. Trousers in solid colours go best with a patterned jacket. Think of matching tones rather than of matching colours. A soft and a hard tone should not be paired, but soft with soft and hard with hard. Grey flannel trousers can be worn with most jacket patterns, beige chinos go well with all sportswear.

TROUSERS

HISTORY

The ancient Persians, the Chinese and the mounted Mongol hordes all waged war in calf-length trousers. Perhaps in consequence of fighting the Persians for so long, the Greeks regarded any form of legged garment as barbaric. It was left to the tribes of northern Europe to introduce trousers to the Romans, who adopted them as cold weather wear for their troops while still frowning upon their use in the capital itself.

Charlemagne, the 9th-century European emperor, wore a form of trouser cross-gartered to the knees and this style endured until the Crusaders brought home new ideas and fabrics, silks and velvets, and trousers were replaced by tight hose. Gentlemen showed their legs for the following 600 years, usually sprouting from breeches which over the centuries fluctuated to fashionable extremes until brought short by the social upheaval that was the French Revolution. The revolutionaries were known as sans-culottes (implying, roughly, 'breechless bums') and the notion of a simpler, classless way of dressing took hold throughout Europe. Tight-fitting pantaloons, named after a character in Italian comedy, were worn from the 1790s and these were shortly followed by the first narrow trousers, inspired by a looser garment worn by sailors.

Americans, eager to assert sartorial as well as political independence, were quickest to abandon the breeches of their colonial past and to this day they refer to trousers as pants, shortened from pantaloon. Pantaloons were almost indistinguishable from trousers when they finally faded out in the course of the 19th century, leaving us with two words for one garment.

As with any radical change in dress, trousers were deemed for some time to be a cause of dissipation.

'Fast talk and slang came in with trousers,' Edward
Bulwer-Lytton maintained.

STYLE

Creases were not generally adopted until the invention of the trouser press in the 1890s, and as late as
1934 George V persisted in having his trousers
creased sideways (in respect for an old navy style)
instead of fore-and-aft like his subjects. Turn-ups,
'cuffs' to the trade, also first became popular in the
1890s, after years of occasional experimentation.

Innumerable legends foster the assumption that
crease and cuff are royal inventions. One of the
most fetching of these tales has the future Edward
VII falling from his horse into a ditch and being
carried into a cottage to rest while his clothes are
dried; in a state of nerves bordering upon panic, the
cottager irons the trousers to a sharp crease and the
surprising result so pleases the prince that he, and
consequently the rest of the world, iron creases into
their trousers from that time forth.

Other stories attribute the invention of the turn-up
to the same clothes-conscious royal, again through
an act of forgetfulness. One version has Edward
turning up the bottoms of his trouser-legs to protect them while crossing a muddy field, then absent-

mindedly returning to London with trousers still
rolled; his loyal subjects take this to be a style indicator and soon the entire world is following suit.
Nothing of the sort ever happened, yet in both
cases royal adoption of a new mode was crucial to
its mass acceptance. In the case of creases, the crucial moment can be pin-pointed to the sensation of
the 1886 Derby, when the elegantly frock-coated
Edward appeared in a pair of grey trousers with
sharply-ironed creases. Turn-ups had a more insidi-
ous aspect to their adoption – the subconscious
notion born of the muddy-field scenario that here
was a city gentleman with interests (i.e. property
and therefore wealth) in the country.

Tradition further credits Edward VII with the
invention of the trouser pleat, again erroneously.
The top-pleat, or fold, was hardly seen until the
beginning of the 20th century, when trousers
became larger and the insertion of pleats con-
tributed to their neater management.

Savile Row tailors were unsettled by this development to the point at which Edward's namesake and
grandson, the future Edward VIII, in the 1920s
denounced in public the baggy, unpleated trousers
of his personal cutter, the mighty Scholte, and
favoured in their place a trimmer American design.

This action exerted a powerful influence on trouser style through the rest of the century.

The same prince was quick to adopt the newfangled zip fastener in place of the buttoned fly, thereby giving the royal nod to this audacious development of the mid-1930s, fifty years after the invention of the zipper.

FIT AND CUT

Creases have by now become so permanent a feature as to be taken for granted, but all else about trousers remains a matter of subtly shifting style and discretionary taste.

Apart from the size of the leg, the cut varies according to whether the waist is set high or low, and whether the trousers are intended to be supported by a belt, or by braces, or by a choice of both. Fit is all-important, to the extent that the wearer's characteristic posture – strut, slouch, or whatever – needs ideally to be studied, and allowances built into the cut

A choice has to be made between having pleats and doing without them. Affording as they do a comfortable, wider cut, pleated trousers set the standard in classic menswear. Pleats anchor the line and facilitate an elegant fall to the garment, even if stressed by hands slung into the pockets. There is a further choice between single and double pleats, and between making the fold inwards or outwards: there is no 'right way.'

Nothing is more subject to 'fashion' excess than the width of the leg. Trim without being tight should always be the objective, with three-quarters the length of the shoe the general rule. As for leg length, the trouser needs to break slightly over the instep of the shoe. Trousers without turn-ups should be cut slightly longer at the back.

True to the rural ambiance of their origin, turn-ups must never be seen on formal wear, since they convey, still, an air of sporty casualness. They should ordinarily rise approximately three to four centimetres. Shorter gentlemen may choose a narrower rise, or dispense with turn-ups altogether.

Side pockets need to be deep, for practical purposes and because this contributes to a smooth line. Button flies have the weight of tradition behind them, but are laborious to attend to. Trousers with zips tend to hang better and crease less.

Quality trousers should come fitted with a half-lining, which contributes to a better drape while improving both comfort and durability.

> FAUX PAS
> Formal suits with turn-ups
> Double-breasted suits without turn-ups
> Casual 'separates' without turn-ups

MATERIAL AND MATCH

The classic pair of grey flannel trousers makes a perfect match for both blazer and tweed jacket. Cotton trousers in solid colours and sports jackets are another traditional combination.

A discreet check combines well with a blazer. Colourful casual trousers goes well with a jersey or blouson.

A remarkable variety of trouser materials work well with the navy blazer. They include flannel, cavalry twill, tropical worsted, linen, and white duck, which though derived from *doek* (Dutch for canvas) is made of cotton.

Cavalry twill, a durable woollen or worsted cloth with a diagonal rib, was as its name implies used primarily for riding wear before being adopted for sports trousers and even two-piece suits. Bedford cord is another excellent trouser material with military antecedents. A sturdy, closely-woven woollen, cotton or blended fabric with a raised cord effect, it was first used to make uniforms for the Bedford Militia, which explains the name.

For all its versatility, flannel has a marked tendency to wear out in zones of friction, in particular in the area of the seat. The effect is most marked in the case of very robust gentlemen, who are best advised to choose other fabrics.

ACCESSORIES

BELT

The belt has always been more than a means of holding things up. Since early times it has been associated with a sense of power and virility. On occasion it has functioned as a mark of rank, never more than in the age of chivalry, when it was the emblem of the knight – richly wrought in precious metals and worn low around the hips.

By the 19th century, the belt had lost all status and was hardly to be seen, except around the midriff of toiling sportsmen. It was American influence, coupled with the eager advocacy of the Prince of Wales, that began to turn attitudes around in the

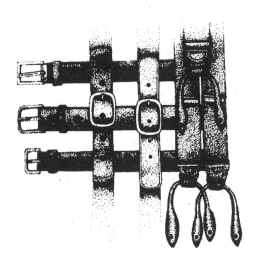

1920s. Belted trousers became increasingly popular with the mass acceptance of the two-piece suit, which in discarding the waistcoat exposed to view frequently ugly braces. By the 1960s, belts had almost wholly supplanted braces, other than in the realm of formal wear, while a prevailing youth fashion rendered them almost as low-slung and ostentatious as those girdles of the knights of yore.

A belt for casual wear may be colourful, and fitted with a striking buckle, so long as not too large or flashy. Exotic leathers such as lizard skin make belts of distinction that border upon presumption. For business suits, a plain belt is strongly recommended.

It must be darker in shade than the suit and should not exceed 3 cm in width. Those who insist upon wearing a belt with evening wear should select one in elegant black calf with a neat silver buckle.

As a general rule, belt and shoes should be similar in colour, though not identical (exception: black). Suede shoes always call for a suede belt.

The tongue of the belt should always extend 5 cm beyond the buckle.

BRACES

The French lay claim to the invention of braces as *bretelles*, strips of ribbon fixed into buttonholes around the time of the Revolution. These were adopted personally by Napoleon, who had his pair decorated with bumblebees, a symbol of his native Corsica.

The idea was generally adopted from the 1820s, as trousers became wider and higher at the waist and required supporting. For more than a century the adjustable, elasticised development of bretelles known as braces ('suspenders' in America) held sway.

As described above, a royal trend-setter conspired with changing times to drive braces to near extinction in the 20th century, before reaction set in with the fuller trousers of the 1990s. This brought blessed relief to the portly and new opportunities to the sartorially savvy.

Braces lost their frumpy image through imaginative new designs, the loudest of which were seized upon by politicians and others who discovered that a bold set of braces seemed to broaden shoulders and narrow the waistline, while hinting at raw power straining at the leash. In consequence, vivid reds wore out their welcome and need to be avoided at all costs.

In choosing between traditional buttoned braces and metal clip-ons, the traditional are much to be preferred. Certain Americans elect to wear braces and a belt at the same time. This has to be avoided at all costs.

FAUX PAS

Wearing braces and a belt at the same time.

TIELOCKEN BURBERRY

Perfect Security With Distinction

The smartness essential in a Top-coat for every-day use, allied to such dependable powers of protection as enable the wearer to face the worst weather without discomfort or risk to health, are universally admitted to be the outstanding characteristics of The Tielocken.

A Double Shield Where Most Needed

Overlapping fronts completely protect all the vulnerable parts of the body, providing, from chin to knees, light, healthful and efficient security against wet and cold.

Proof Without Enervating Heat

Burberry proofing, whilst rendering the materials non-absorbent, satisfies every hygienic condition. Unlike rubber-proofed cloths or oiled-silk linings, it allows self-ventilation, and entirely obviates the unhealthy heat engendered by these air-tight fabrics.

No Buttons To Fasten or Lose

Another valuable feature of The Tielocken is its easy adjustment. All buttons are avoided, and with the exception of the upright collar, the coat is securely held by a smart belt.

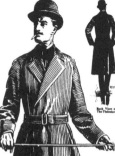

Back View of The Tielocken

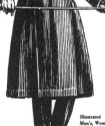

Illustrated Men's, Women's and Military Catalogues Post Free.

Burberry copyright

The Tielocken Burberry

"*Tielocken coats provide double protection over the vital parts of the body where it is most needed, the overlapping fronts keeping the chest and legs safeguarded against bitingly cold winds or driving rain.*

"*There is no possibility of these fronts blowing open and letting in unwelcome draughts and damp, and so the Tielocken models are the most perfectly protective wraps imaginable.*" —BADMINTON MAGAZINE.

Every Burberry Garment is labelled "Burberrys"

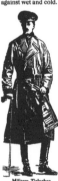

Military Tielocken

"*This coat is as comfortable that I shall be sorry when it is worn out. It is the best protection against wind and rain that I have ever met.*" —H.S.

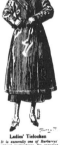

Ladies' Tielocken

"*It is assuredly one of Burberrys happiest inspirations for ensuring protection, freedom and comfort in any season and in any weather*" —LADIES' FIELD.

BURBERRYS   Haymarket S.W. LONDON
Bd. Malesherbes PARIS: and Provincial Agents

OVERCOATS

HISTORY

The overcoat, commonly referred to as simply the coat, can be traced back to the 17th century. Prior to that, outer protective garments consisted of untailored mantels, such as cloaks or capes. Ancient Britons made do with a piece of cloth which doubled as a mantle by day and a blanket at night. The fabric with which it was made has come down to us in the form of Scottish and Irish plaids.

The Roman toga was as much as 5.5 metres long and more than 2.1 metres wide and must have required assistance to drape in the stately manner prescribed. This was too much for most people, and by later Roman times they were wearing outer garments in use to this day in the form of such sacred Christian vestments as the chausible, which as the casula was an everyday mantle, or poncho, dropping easily over the shoulders, with an opening for the head to pop through.

Cloaks with sleeves did not appear until 16th century, initially for riding. The buff (from 'buffalo') coat of leather was a military overgarment widely popular in the 17th century, while a long, loose outer garment with cuffed sleeves and open side seams for the sword to hang through was very fashionable by the 1660s.

When, in the 18th century, the riding coat became adapted for genteel indoor wear, a similar but much bulkier 'greatcoat', or surtout, was introduced, with full skirts and centre-vent, the latter being required to accommodate the back of a horse. By the 1790s, the greatcoat had acquired deep overlapping collars. As the Carrick, it reached almost to the ground and became familiar throughout Europe as the wear of coachmen.

The early decades of the 19th century saw greatcoats become so modish that they were being worn whatever the weather. In 1830, the author of a book on sartorial style declared that no 'fashionable' man would be seen without his black, blue or olive 'surtout-coat', with pinched waist, full skirt, and puffed-up, velvet-lapelled chest.

The surtout gave way to the Paletot, an abbreviated greatcoat, but soon a term covering overcoats in general. Styles proliferated in confused abundance, most soon to be forgotten, but a few destined to become classics.

The Chesterfield appeared first as a development of the frock coat, evolving gradually over the century into the classic formal overcoat. The Inverness Cape, a wide-sleeved tweed overcoat with shoulder-cape, was a favourite of Victorian travellers. The Ulster was a heavy tweed overcoat, full and belted, with a detachable hood, introduced by a Belfast firm in the 1860s. Thirty years later, the *Tailor and Cutter* advised that "no gentleman's wardrobe is complete without an Ulster".

The trade journal was for technical reasons less enthusiastic about the distinctive, slope-shouldered Raglan, finding it "somewhat difficult to cut", but that did limit the popularity of this light and adaptable style dating from the time of the Crimean War. By the 1890s, there were Raglans made of fabric which had been water-proofed.

The smell of soggy woollen greatcoats is alone sufficient to explain why effective waterproofing so exercised 19th-century minds. Cloth treated with oil – oilskin – was a kind of solution and enthusiasts took to boiling clothing for hours in oily concoctions of their own invention in attempts to make it impermeable. In 1823, the Scottish chemist Charles Macintosh patented his method of bonding rubber between layers of cloth, and within a few years waterproof cloak and cape 'macintoshes' were being produced, but they were stiff, smelly and potentially unhealthy.

Enter Thomas Burberry, a country draper who recognised that the solution demanded a material which allowed free passage of air even while excluding water. After much experiment, he hit upon a method of chemically treating cotton fabric so that it repelled water while remaining porous. Burberry moved to London in 1891 and became world famous, first for his ingenious all-conditions sportswear, proclaimed in an advertisement of 1904 to be "PROOF against the Heaviest Rains and Mists, the Stoutest Thorn or Fishhook', and then for his raincoat".

The overcoat, a military innovation at the outset, was hugely influential in, and influenced by, the great wars of the 20th century. The singular demands of trench warfare were answered by the British Warm, a short, comfortable double-breasted officer's coat that replaced a standard-issue greatcoat. It was joined by the rain-resistant cotton gabardine trenchcoat, designed by Burberry's uniform department and issued to more than half a million men in the course of the war.

Both these coats went on to post-war glory; the British Warm in slightly adapted form, the trench-coat with all of its militaristic panache and para-phernalia intact. The hooded, durable Duffle coat, at first a Royal Navy garment dubbed the convoy coat, became the signature-wear of Field-Marshall Montgomery in the Second World War and without quite achieving the enduring impact of those other war-coats it proved immensely popular when launched commercially in the early 1950s.

The motor car and other phenomena of 20th-century living had a influence on outerwear of all kinds. Early needs of the open roadster dictated that the 'motoring coat' be brutishly big and belted and usually of leather because, as the *Tailor and Cutter* put it, "when travelling at a high rate of speed, the ordinary cloth is not sufficient protection for the chest". With the enclosed and ever more comfort-able 'saloon' car came a drastically different set of requirements, for a coat that was easy to put on and off, and slight enough not to hamper driving.

With ceaseless advances in man-made fibres cou-pling with new ideas in abbreviated car coats, anoraks and windcheaters, style was often to suffer in the scramble for clever novelty.

MATERIAL

Heavier milled woollen cloths, such as melton, cheviot and the tweeds are traditional for overcoats, with the choice depending upon both style and occasion. While overcoats of cashmere or vicuna are gorgeous to wear, they are not nearly as sturdy as those made of sheep's wool. For this reason, fabric mixtures are often preferred. The same goes for the camel-hair coat.

WOOL

Wool is a most satisfactory coating material. The natural fat content makes it water-repellent and its capacity to provide warmth is not lessened by damp conditions.

CASHMERE

A particularly soft and warm coating, combed out of Asian goats. Not very hard wearing.

VICUNA

This very rare and valuable undercoat of a high Andes relative of the llama has been called the wool of kings. If your tastes are royal, indulge yourself, but be aware that it is fragile.

CAMEL HAIR

The tan-to-brown fur from the thick, soft under-coat of the Bactrian camel is extremely practical and durable.

TWEED

This rough-textured woollen fabric of irregular woollen yarns in many patterns makes a practical, warm coating material. Harris tweed is spun, dyed and woven by crofters of Scotland's Western Isles.

SHETLAND

A warm and light mixed-colour wool with a heavy nap. Softer and finer than Harris tweed, it will not take heavy wear at the elbows and cuffs and is for those who value character in the sportswear. This homespun comes from islands to the north of the Scottish mainland. Similar wools from elsewhere that are woven in the same manner are properly called 'Shetland-wool types'.

LODEN

A light and very warm fabric that is naturally water-repellent due to the high fat content of the type of wool used. First made in the Tyrolean Alps, where it was named after the *ëlodererí*, or weaver. Tradition dictates that it should be in green.

DONEGAL
A tweed first woven by crofters in County Donegal, Ireland. It is distinguished by its knobbly structure.

MELTON
Heavy, slightly fuzzed overcoat fabric, first worn by huntsmen from Melton Mowbray in England. Fleece coating is similar to Melton in having a napped surface.

HERRINGBONE
The name aptly describes the fine, zigzag pattern of this ribbed twill fabric whose threads slant right and left like the bones of a fish.

COTTON
Various finishing processes enable cotton to be used as a coating. Distinctively ribbed cotton-poplin once mercerised and treated to resist water, makes an easy-care raincoat material.

DOUBLE FACE
A substantial material composed of two layers of fabric bound together; ideal for winter overcoats. The fabrics may differ, with either side used as the face.

COLOURS

The more formal the occasion, the darker the hue. The Chesterfield expresses its dignity in dark grey, blue, or black of course.

Navy and camel are traditional for town coats, though both suffer from a tendency to look scruffy after comparatively light soiling. Sports coats are often in tweed, whose grainy patterns harmonise with their informality. A black and white herring-bone and a Donegal in mixed earthy hues are other deservedly popular styles.

Raincoats are traditionally in beige, green and brown. The classic stone trenchcoat is felt to mature with wear, though one must be vigilant that 'character' does not become a polite interpretation of grubbiness. For country wear, blue or green works better than stone.

STYLE

One must never forget that the prime purpose of any overcoat is to protect the wearer from inclement weather. This said, there is no reason to sacrifice style for practicality. A good coat should look good, whether it be a simple raincoat or a venerable Chesterfield.

The cosseted, centrally-heated modern lifestyle has reduced our call upon overcoats, and one observes a tendency to skimp – perhaps to make do with something 'all-purpose', which, alas, does not quite fit any purpose. While there is no call to go to the other extreme, the gentleman should allow himself a choice of at least two pieces of quality outerwear of a contrasting nature.

As with suits, double-breasted overcoats have peaked lapels, whereas single-breasted have notched lapels.

In determining the right fit of overcoat, it is essential to wear to the fitting room a jacket, or else a heavy pullover.

The coat should ordinarily reach beyond the knees, both for the sake of a good line and because anything less tends to suffer the crumples when sat upon. The sleeves should cover both the jacket and the shirt sleeves. Gentlemen with low centres of gravity need to beware of a single back vent which rises high enough to enter the zone of maximum stress.

HAVELOCK

This sleeveless, hip-length cape coat of black woollen fabric is still worn over the tailcoat to complete a classic formal ensemble. It is named after a British general who died in 1857.

CHESTERFIELD

This classic plain-back, slightly-shaped overcoat makes its presence felt through simple elegance. It has flap pockets and a breast welt pocket. It may have a single-breasted fly (concealed) front, or be double-breasted. The velvet collar is optional. It takes its name from a 19th-century Earl of Chesterfield.

BRITISH WARM

The military background of this snappy overcoat is clearly visible. Two rows of buttons, slightly shaped body lines, slanting flap pockets and (usually) epaulets all reflect the original design for officers in the Great War. Double-breasted, in knee or above-knee length, it may be made of fleece or melton cloth.

Raglan

This popular, loose-fitting overcoat without shoulder seams has full-cut sleeves running up to the neck. It is generally buttoned through, with notched lapels and cuff straps. It is named after Lord Raglan, heroic bungler of the Crimean War, and thereupon hangs a tale, or two.

One version has Lord Raglan keeping warm in the frigid Balaclava winter by cutting a hole for his head in a service blanket, thereby incidentally inventing what became the Raglan cut. This sounds unlikely for a man obsessed with plumed splendour. Let us rather heed an alternative yarn – that he had his tailor design a coat sleeve to disguise as much as possible his loss of an arm in battle.

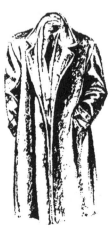

LODEN

A double-breasted overcoat of loden cloth, with a front and back yoke. Light, warm and showerproof, it has become popular for both town and country wear. It may be buttoned or have a wood-toggle closure. The cut usually features an unstitched part of the armhole to provide extra room for manoeuvre.

POLO COAT

A modern American classic that owes everything to its British heritage. This costly camel-hair coat is double-breasted and has patch pockets, cuffs, and a half-belt. It is said to trace its ancestry to the Edwardian polo fields, when sporting gentlemen had their tailors come up with something to throw over their shoulders between chukkers. The result was a so-called 'wait coat', warm but with a certain swagger, which caught the attention of the Gatsby set when rich Americans took up polo in the 1920s. The upshot of this was the 'polo' coat, so imbued with casual elegance that some men are said to be able to carry it off with evening dress.

DUFFLE COAT

This is a square-tailed, three-quarter length coat with hood, made of heavy woollen cloth. A yoke, patch pockets and toggle fastening are its main features. The name comes from Duffel, a Belgian town long associated with hard-wearing woollen fabric.

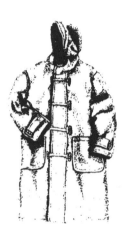

RAINWEAR

Raincoats should be separated into two categories — the truly waterproof, and those that are 'rainproof' or 'showerproof'.

Waterproof implies the use of rubberized materials. When it comes to the second category, there are many methods of making a fabric rain-resistant or water-repellent. They include immersion in a chemical solution, spraying, or applications of oil or wax.

There is a vast selection of rainwear to suit every taste and purpose. Regrettably, gentlemen do not always give this due consideration. A double-textured macintosh, for instance, is practical for winter pursuits, or for a very wet climate, but it is not ideal for sultry conditions or the heat of summer.

A detachable lining, of plaid or fur, will greatly extend a coat's range of effective service.

In selecting a size, one should always allow for plenty of 'room'. A raincoat should be slightly longer than a normal overcoat.

THE TRENCHCOAT

This dashing and yet practical and durable double-breasted all-weather coat comes battle-ready. This is a garment of heroes and of secret agents.

It is double-breasted in water-repellent tightly woven cotton, with epaulets, wrist straps, gun flap and back yoke, spymaster collar and throat latch. The reinforced belt comes with metal D-rings for attaching water bottle and hand grenades, or, if you will, an umbrella...

Could Bogard have endured the loss of Ingrid Bergman and the prospect of going on alone to Casablanca, had he been without his trenchcoat and fedora? Undoubtedly not.

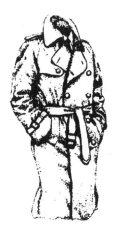

SLIP-ON

This is a single-breasted raincoat. It may have Raglan or set-in sleeves (sleeves sewn in at the armpit) and can have concealed 'fly-front' buttons or be a standard button-through. The cut must be wide and comfortable, with slit pockets for the hands to reach through, two large inside pockets, and adjustable cuff straps.

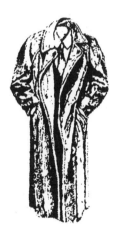

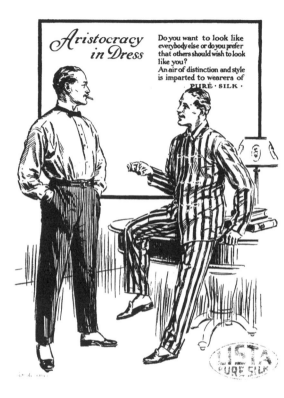

SHIRTS

HISTORY

The shirt is the most basic garment — a protective second skin. For untold centuries it was a loose-fitting tunic, invariably of linen, a cloth used in clothing for at least 10,000 years. As such it has entered the human psyche. To lose the shirt off one's back is to lose all; to wash one's dirty linen in public is to expose all.

Until comparatively recent advances in the growing and processing of cotton, linen provided by far the most practical screen between outerwear and the secretions and sensitivities of the body. It is pliant, soft, absorbent, hard-wearing, and it washes well. The ancient Egyptians revelled in it, and after death were wrapped up in it.

Silk, by comparison, was too delicate and too expensive for all but a privileged few. In the colder climates of northern Europe, some early shirts were made of wool, but wool does not pass the wash-test well. Cotton, until well into the 19th century, was beneath contempt, considered useful only for padding and stuffing.

The word shirt has been traced to an early Germanic word meaning short: the same root that has given us 'skirt'. For most of its history, the shirt was a very basic T-shaped tunic made of cloth taken straight from the loom and requiring no tailoring skills. Until the middle of the 19th century it was made at home by hand, usually by the wife or some servant.

Size and fit were of no consequence – plenty of billowing linen was a proclamation of wealth – with the sole proviso that it had to be of sufficient length to protect the neck and wrists from chafing on the edges of the outer garments. Eureka: the collar and cuffs, peek-a-boo elements which gave the shirt enticement value as the piece of underwear which exposed itself.

Fancy collars and cuffs were an inevitable development, leading in the Elizabethan age to the extravagant excesses of the ruff. This vast, radiating neckband of linen trimmed with lace was starched until it stuck out all around like a cartwheel. Ruffs were gradually allowed to collapse back on the shoulders, but the crisp effect of starch upon linen would be returned to again and again.

Lace and ruffle were abandoned by the end of the 18th century, replaced by expanses of white linen under the general supervision of Beau Brummell, whose motto was "fine linen, plenty of it, and country washing".

Simplicity was married to sophistication: the finer, the softer, the whiter the linen, the greater the distinction. Since white linen shows up the slightest speck of dirt, it was a cruelly effective way of excluding from social contention all but those rich enough, and idle enough, to be able to change their shirts several times a day.

A compromise of sorts was found in the detached starched collar, which for a century held the new professional classes in throttled thraldom. In one of these unverifiable stories which so decorate the history of dress, a Mrs. Hannah Montague is a claimant to its invention. It seems that Mrs. Montague so resented washing shirts that one morning in 1820 she snipped off her husband's collars to minimise the daily drudgery.

The tight starched collar, or choker, evolved in hundreds of styles, of which the wing collar, with points folded back from the throat, was welcomed for at least offering some degree of relief. The 'boiled shirt' with wing collar was the only way to dress up properly. It had to be boiled to remove the stiff starch of its front panel, hence the name.

The boiled shirt was, of course, of linen. Cotton shirting consisted only of cheap calicoes worn by labourers, though through the latter part of the 19th century some striped cottons were seen at recreational events. The double, or turned-down style of the modern collar began to come into use in the second half of the 19th century, but only with casual clothes.

In 1900, an American shirt manufacturer tested the limits of sex appeal in starch when it created the stiff-necked Arrow Collar Man as a hunk of male magnificence… "languorous of lid, the eyes piercing, the chin noble, the mouth innocent. Overall, an air of calm". The sales response to this marketing ploy was phenomenal, but soft shirts were by now becoming available in variety in America. Another American innovation about this time was the modern style of 'coat' shirt, which buttoned all the way down the front and hence did not require to be pulled over the head.

Starch had become so associated with male dignity that it was hard to dispense with, but the Great War generation had the starch knocked out of it in every sense, and in the new Prince of Wales it found a style leader who was no stuffed shirt either. By the 1930s, the prince was wearing soft shirts even with his dinner clothes.

Poplins and other cottons were now becoming really popular and shirts were coming with built-in 'stiffeners' to ease a gradual transition back to the soft attached collar.

F. Scott Fitzgerald captured the hedonism of the new freedom to self-indulge in this unparalleled description from *The Great Gatsby*:

"He took out a pile of shirts and began throwing them, one by one, before us, shirts of sheer linen and thick silk and fine flannel, which lost their folds as they fell and covered the table in many-coloured disarray. While we admired, he brought more and the soft rich heap mounted higher — shirts with stripes and scrolls and plaids in coral and apple-green and lavender and faint orange, with monograms of Indian blue. Suddenly, with a strained sound, Daisy bent her head into the shirts and began to cry stormily. 'They're such beautiful shirts,' she sobbed, her voice muffled in the thick folds. 'It makes me sad because I've never seen such — such beautiful shirts before.'"

MATERIALS

COTTON-BATISTE
This finely-woven fabric is thin enough to be semi-transparent. It is thought to be named after Baptiste of Cambrai, a French linen weaver of legendary accomplishment.

COTTON-POPLIN
A shirting fabric with a slight ribbed effect achieved in the warp. Some of the best poplins are known as 'sea island', after a variety of particularly long-staple cotton originating in Egypt and grown on islands off the south-east coast of the United States and in the Caribbean. As with batiste, a finishing treatment with a solution of caustic soda adds to its strength and lustre. This process is known as mercerising. It was developed in 1844 by an English calico printer named John Mercer.

OXFORD
A coloured-woven cotton fabric in plain or basket weave that is often used for hard-wearing sports shirts.

HARVARD

Coloured-woven cloth with a twill weave and colour effects similar to that of Oxford cotton.

FLANNELETTE (COTTON-FLANNEL)

This cotton shirting material is napped – furred – by a milling process to achieve a soft surface texture on either side. The result is a warm fabric that mimics all-wool flannel.

CHAMBRAY

A woven cotton with a coloured warp and white weft filling. It is used to make a fine jeans shirt fabric.

LINEN

This was universal shirt fabric until replaced by cotton, which is easier and cheaper to raise. It is stronger and more absorbent than cotton and its crisp appearance and cool feel make it ideal for summer shirts. Linen's notorious wrinkliness can be corrected by impregnating the fibres with a crease-resistant resin.

SILK

Silk makes a most comfortable and luxurious shirt fabric. Silk shirtings range from coarse and nubby Shantung, made from the wild 'tussah' silk of cocoons gathered in China and India, to the fine gauze-like crêpe de Chine.

WOOL

Woollen shirts are manufactured from fine worsteds. There are also quality blends, such as wool/cashmere, wool/silk, wool/cotton (Viyella is a branded wool-cotton blend). Flannel shirts are also made of wool.

INTERLOCK

The close-knit fabric of polo shirts and T-shirts is created through this process. Machines with alternating short and long needles form a mesh-like material of high elasticity. Such knitted fabrics are highly elastic despite maintaining their shape.

PATTERNS

PLAIN

Classic white remains the mark of the gentleman. The terminology relating to white and blue collar dates from the 19th century, when the white collar distinguished the clerk from the manual worker, whose circumstances obliged him to dress in blue or some other colour to hide the inevitable dirt. Though, in point of fact, manual workers in those days tended to wear no collar at all.

Nowadays every colour imaginable may be employed on business shirts, so long as the tone is sufficiently muted. Tones for sports shirts can be a shade richer.

STRIPES

Striped sports shirts, popularly known as regatta shirts, became popular in the 1870s. Equipped with white collar and cuffs, they have since ascended to the heights of sartorial classicism, as witness the way they are worn by modern American dandy Tom Wolfe.

BENGAL STRIPE

Colourful, striped fabric that originated in India.

END-TO-END

A cotton twill fabric with small patterns in the form of stairs. The warp threads, known as 'ends', alternate between a light and a dark colour.

MADRAS

This plain-weave cotton fabric has something of the appearance of end-to-end. It can also be in twill weave. Like many cotton fabrics, it originated in India.

TATTERSALL

Checked pattern of vertical and horizontal stripes, usually in two colours upon a light background. It is named after an 18th-century London horse market where sportsmen forgathered wearing waistcoats of this pattern.

VICHY CHECK

A two-coloured pattern of small checks popularised in the 1960s. It is more identified with cravats than with the necktie.

FANCIES

This term embraces all manner of striking designs for sports and leisure shirts, from tropical Hawaiian prints to paisley patterns.

COLLAR TYPES

Collar flaps are known as 'points' and the space between them is the 'spread'. Today there are about a half-dozen common variations of the regular collar type, plus one dignified throwback to more formal times.

TURN-DOWN COLLAR

This is the regular collar. It comes in various forms and sizes, from short and wide to long and slim. The version sometimes known as the short point is the standard collar for business wear and the most versatile, being appropriate to most occasions.

WING COLLAR

A stand-up collar with folded-back points (the wings) that is correct for formal wear with a tail-coat, dinner jacket or morning coat.

TAB COLLAR

The collar points, which may be pointed or rounded, are constricted by means of a buttoned tab hidden under the tie-knot.

PIN COLLAR

The pin collar, again either pointed or round, achieves much the same effect as the tab collar, while affording the wearer an opportunity to discreetly display an item of jewellery. The collar is equipped with holes for attaching the gold collar pin.

BUTTON-DOWN COLLAR

The collar points are held in place by a button to the shirt. This is the jauntiest collar that one can wear to the office. It is extremely adaptable, being able to take a full windsor knot, or a bow tie for that matter.

A fanciful tale traces its origin to the ingenuity of British polo players irritated by their collars flying in the wind, but this most American of styles is better sourced across the Atlantic among Ivy League students of the 1920s. The button-down look combines nonchalance with precision to create an air of confident, easy-going efficiency that goes down well in the modern business world, hence its popularity.

FIT

COLLAR

A few simple rules need to be observed. Gentlemen with long necks should select high collars; those with full necks are advised to chose shallower collars. Care should be taken that the collar is not too tight.

To correctly assess collar size, hold one end of a tape measure to the throat by the collar button and let it loosely surround the neck, allowing sufficient room for movement.

SLEEVES AND CUFFS

The sleeve length is measured from the centre of the back yoke to the end of the cuff. Cuffs should fit closely while leaving room for movement. At least 1 cm of the cuff should be visible underneath the suit sleeve.

WAIST

This is a matter of personal discretion. One should note that tight, body-hugging shirts were a happening of the 1960s, intriguingly the only time in history when there has been such a vogue.

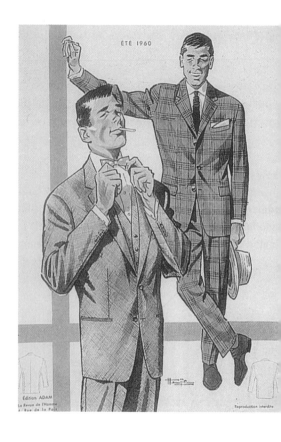

ÉTÉ 1960

Ties

History

Strictly speaking, the modern tie was a Victorian invention, though it is impossible to be precise about the evolution of the ribbon that gentlemen wear around their necks.

"Did the Greeks and Romans wear collars and ties, and if not, why not?" the clothes connoisseur James Laver has pondered with a smile.

Neckclothes, as distinct from ties, can be traced to antiquity. The troops of the Chinese emperor who began building the Great Wall wore a kind of neck-wear, and Roman soldiers had their sudaria, a muslin cloth to absorb perspiration on the march. This was not to be confused with the focalia, a woolly neck-cloth that Roman orators used to protect their vocal chords in chilly weather. The Emperor Augustus wore one of those, though only at home; it was not the kind of thing an Emperor wished to be seen wearing in public.

Achieving general agreement on what was presentable took a further 1600 years. The details of how it came about are in dispute. What is certain is that collars, then known as 'bands', were the sole focus of interest until they culminated in the cartwheel Elizabethan ruff. Detumescence thereupon set in with a 'falling band' of frilly lace, which in the reign of Charles II began to be kept in place by something quite new called a 'cravat'.

The word cravat may or may not derive from the French word for Croat, but Francophiles and romantics in general hold that in Croatia, which was a remote corner of the Roman Empire, the ancient forms of neckwear survived the millennia to be worn by Croatian mercenaries fighting with the French in the Thirty Years War. The French officers liked the jaunty air of the soldiers' neck-cloths, so the story goes, and so did their king, that great fashion plate Louis XIV.

Louis appointed a master cravatier, established a light cavalry regiment called the Royal Cravates, and equipped his forces with silk cravats. Every morning, the royal cravatier would present the king with a basketful of cravats, decorated with ribbons of crimson, scarlet, orange and pale blue. The king would chose one, tie the knot himself, and leave the arrangement to the cravatier.

So ends the pretty tale. Other authorities argue that Louis had little or nothing to do with it: that the cravat had already evolved in England from satin and velvet ribbons that held together a 'crabbat', or neck frill.

Whatever the truth, the style spread quickly. In 1660, the first cravat reached America, ordered from England for £5 by the Governor of Virginia. If this sounds expensive for the time, Charles II's successor, James II, paid £36 and ten shillings for a cravat of Venice lace to wear at his coronation in 1685.

The cravat could be worn in many ways – with coloured ribbons, or in a bow under the chin, or loosely knotted. In 1692, English troops surprised the French near Steinkirk in Belgium and shortly thereafter a style 'a la Steinkerque' became the rage. This involved twisting the long ends together and using a buttonhole as anchor, which is what the French troops are imagined to have done in their haste to get to battle.

Before all of these styles could be sorted out, the loose cravat gave way to the stock, which was a tight neck-band of folded linen, sometimes stiffened with horsehair or whalebone. Stocks were worn from the 1730s and they still are today in a modified version with hunt uniform.

In the 'solitaire', a black ribboned bow which could be worn over the stock, we have a precursor of the formal 'black tie', but in the 1780s the cravat was back in favour. It consisted now of a large square of linen which was doubled into a triangle, then folded over and over before being passed round and sometimes round and round the neck and then knotted or tied in a bow.

The cravat was required to nestle in such a manner that the upright points of the starched shirt collar showed just above its top edge, thereby all but encasing the lower jaw. Pristine white and lightly starched, it became the object of more fuss than any other item in sartorial history.

The peerless Beau Brummell was prepared to invest an entire morning in quest of the perfect swathing and the perfect knot. The story is told of a visitor calling upon the beau and finding himself knee-deep in crumpled linen. "Sir," said the valet, "these are our failures."

Lesser interpreters could get themselves into dire straits. Dickens writes of a character throttling himself to the point where 'I almost believe I saw creases come into the whites of his eyes.'

It was all too much to sustain, if not to bear. By the 1830s, the blinding billows of white starch were a memory, to be persevered only in the starched white fronts of evening dress. Loosely-knotted scarfs were affected for a time and these took many forms; one style, dubbed the 'Byron', was narrow enough to pass for a string tie.

Around mid-century we at last come upon the term 'necktie'. The cravat was by now being wound around the neck once and tied in front with a very large and often loud-coloured bow (from whence, the 'bow tie') or else it was tightly knotted at the throat to leave long ends dangling down the shirt-front (from whence the standard modern tie), or it was fold-ed across the chest and fixed with a pin in a style which would become the ascot. That dubious item, the 'made-up' bow tie, also made its début in the 1860s.

It so chanced that the knot-and-dangle version provided an ideal focal point for a new kind of 'lounging' jacket with V-opening at the chest, and together they proceeded to conquer the entire world, as suit and tie. The phenomenon happened so swift-ly that the conquest was all but complete by 1900.

Major design advances occurred in the 1920s, when an American tie manufacturer named Jesse Langsdorf pioneered a construction method which enabled the tie to snap back into shape after knotting. This featured the use of loose stitching and a bias-cut wool interlining, where previously flannel had been used. By the 1930s, quality ties were being expertly cut, always on the cross grain of the fabric to achieve maximum resilience.

SHAPES AND KNOTS

Oscar Wilde said it: "A well-tied tie is the first serious step in life." Since early in the 19th century, the quest for the perfect knot has been the cause of unremitting effort and ingenuity.

At the height of the cravat obsession, there were at least 100 recognisable knots, including the Gordian Knot, so complicated that the wearer could be extracted only with shears or scissors. The French novelist Honoré de Balzac is said to have been the mysterious H. le Blanc whose best-selling instructional manual detailed the ins and outs of 32 of them, with names like the Napoleon, the Oriental, and the Mail Coach.

The Mail Coach may have had something to do with the naming of the Four-in-Hand, the basic tie-knot of today. The four-in-hand is named after the manner in which coachmen controlled the reins of a team of horses. Slim and asymmetrical, it is distinguished by a little dimple immediately beneath the knot.

The Windsor knot dates from the 1930s and is named for the Duke of Windsor, who then favoured large knots. Symmetrical, bulky and triangular, it is tied in a special manner with extra loops.

The bow tie is a subject on its own. Never out of fashion, and of course an essential part of formal evening wear, it nevertheless comes under suspicion from elements who regard its everyday use as an affectation of the eccentric. Some of this suspicion may mask embarrassment from not knowing how to handle a bow tie; in particular, how to tie it. This is easier than it appears, being much like tying one's shoelaces.

A permanently tied bow is wholly lacking in style, and is impossible to disguise. A gentleman must therefore persevere and learn to tie his own: one can practise on the thigh, or on the arm of a chair. Bow ties are commonly of silk or barathea, silk being the more difficult to tie.

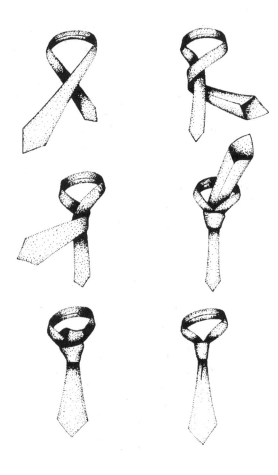

The asymmetrical, simple four-in-hand knot

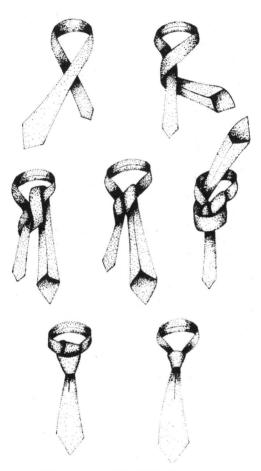

The symmetrical half-Windsor knot

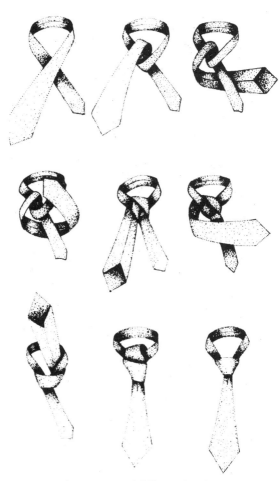

The symmetrical full-Windsor knot

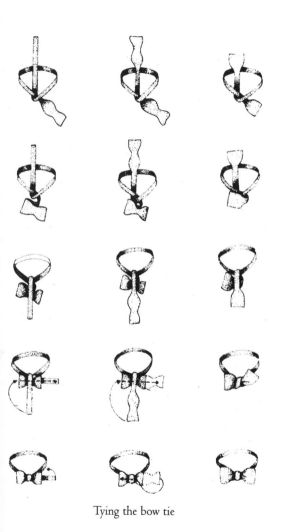

Tying the bow tie

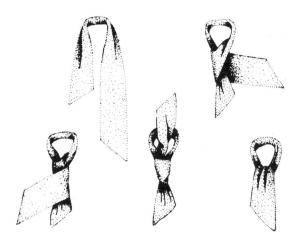

Tying a scarf tie

Neck-scarfs or cravats are tied in simple knots. The ascot normally comes cut in its Edwardian mode, with a narrow, pleated centre section to negotiate the collar, and wider ends for puffing up in the shirt opening. An intriguing alternative is to be your own Beau Brummell. A large silk square folded to form a triangle, then fold-rolled to an appropriate width, can be knotted and tucked as one chooses. The Duke of Windsor achieved a simple elegance just by threading the ends through a finger-ring.

MATERIALS AND PATTERNS

The silk tie is above praise or criticism. It is simply the classic mode of neckwear. But please let it be of pure silk, no synthetics.

SILK adorns as no other material can, and it is supple, soft, durable and strong. The wealth of gleaming colours, shades and designs attainable is without equal. Patterns in silk rep are always woven, never printed. This is made possible by an adaptation of the jacquard loom, first used to weave ties with small club emblems in the 1920s. Sports club colours and the long modern necktie were made for each other in every sense, having been twinned since the emergence of the true tie in 1867. The Old School Tie came into general use from the 1890s.

CRÊPE DE CHINE is made of finely twisted silk yarns which give it a crinkled, luminous effect. Such ties can have printed designs or solid colours and go well with flannel or mohair. Some of the more extravagant ties of the 1960s Peacock Revolution were made of this material.

GUM TWILL (foulard) is a lightweight silk twill with a particularly luxurious feel. It is steeped in tradition. The small printed designs are by custom of the 'paisley' type, from an Indian design originally hand-pressed onto the silk with 'madder' dye from a tree root. Gum twill ties may accompany lighter-weight suits or sports jackets.

IRISH POPLIN, in its original form as a superior silk-wool blend, has a long and fascinating story. The name poplin comes from papalina, Italian for papal, and reflects its origins in Avignon, the French town that was for centuries under the rule of the Popes. In 1685, religious persecution drove hundreds of thousands of Huguenots out of France. Among them were numbers of silk weavers who settled in Ireland, where they resumed their labours to good effect.

Irish poplin consists of a silk warp shot through with a worsted weft. The much thicker woollen threads give a firm 'backbone' to the tie, which has a corded, silken surface. Due to the wool content, the material is less prone to curl than pure silk, but it does not take a drenching very well.

WOOL ties come in a variety of mixtures and can contain alpaca or cashmere as well as ordinary wool. They are softer than silk and are suitable for sports jackets, suits made from coarse fabric, and V-neck sweaters.

Knit ties made of silk, wool or alpaca are appropriate for casual wear. They are commonly in solid colours, or stripes. Crocheted ties have been out of favour since the 1960s.

MANUFACTURING

The finest ties are unique, each one a creation unto itself, the product of meticulous craftsmanship extended over 40 separate operations. The quality of the silk and precision of the cut, the quality and cut of the lining, the accuracy of the stitching, all play their part. This needs to be appreciated when reflecting upon the cost of such an item.

CUT

The tie fabric has to be cut on the bias, in other words diagonal to the grain of the weave, at a 45-degree angle to the selvage, or straight edge of the material. This makes for flexibility and ease in tying the knot, and the maintenance of shape. Economising on the material, or cutting the fabric at a slighter angle, would result in the tie losing its straight fall and quickly becoming warped with wear.

Jacquard fabrics — woven on a pattern-control loom — have to be cut individually to ensure that the pattern motifs do not coincide with the tie ends, since this heightens the risk of their fraying out. Individual cutting also guarantees the precise placing of striped patterns: a detail which the connoisseur will appreciate. (The cloth for mass-produced ties is prepared on machines that slice through more than 100 layers at a time.)

The tie begins in two pieces, which are hemmed on the bias in one of the few mechanical operations in hand-made neckwear. The joint at the neck, or piecing, is pressed flat to eliminate neckband bulk where it would inconvenience the wearer.

LINING

Good lining, expertly cut, is the foundation of the superior necktie. It should be of pure wool cut on the bias. Apart from providing a firm foundation, it ensures that the tie retains its shape.

A guage is used to lay in the lining with the necessary precision. The silk 'shell' is then wrapped around the lining and pinned in place every few inches, in an operation comparable to basting in tailoring. Ties made of very thin, very fine silk, such as crêpe de Chine, are fully interlined with pure silk, otherwise the lining would show through.

THE SLIP-STITCH

In this crucial operation, the main seam which forms the tube of the tie is completed by hand. Resilient construction is dependent upon loose, even stitching. The slip-stitch, as it is called, is sewn firmly onto the front and loose at the back to maintain elasticity. This is a little masterpiece of artistry.

A form is inserted to ensure precisely shaped ends. Pressing is done by hand, to avoid a flat, dead look.

STYLE

It has been said of the tie that it is the flag we hoist to signal who we are: that it expresses, just as it gives away, more than any other element of dress. Hence the agony of indecision with which selection is so often associated.

A little planning is in order. Gentlemen have a regrettable tendency to collect ties, old ties being like old teddy bears and not to be abandoned. Far better to have and to care for a select few of top-quality, hand-finished. They should include plain and patterned silks in a careful choice of rich shades, and traditional 'regimental' stripes if you will, though no gentleman should fly under false colours: the *Book of Public School, Old Boys, University, Navy, Army, Air Force & Club Ties* lists and illustrates 749 of the more distinguished!

Avoid ties that clamour for attention. The tie must not be allowed to dominate; nor dare it be a shrinking violet, fading in the face of the shirt. Rather, it must provide a focus for the entire ensemble – the top note in a harmonised symphony. It must therefore be chosen with particularly careful regard to the shirt.

A silk neck-scarf or cravat provides a touch of romance and elegant flamboyance and is a recommended addition.

FAUX PAS
Gum twill tie with a blazer or formal wear
Black bow tie with a tail coat
Standard tie with wing collar
Loosened tie with undone collar

KNITWEAR

HISTORY

Knitting might be said to have been invented by whoever first fashioned a cat's cradle or fishing net. This puts its origins back to the Stone Age, or earlier.

Knitting is the process of producing fabric by interlocking loops of yarn or thread, as distinct from the interlacing process that is weaving. Whereas weaving looms have existed since prehistoric times, the first advance beyond knitting by hand was not achieved until 1589, when a Cambridge divine named William Lee invented a contraption to knit his socks.

A ribbing device followed in 1758 and a warp-knitting machine in 1775, but there was no major improvement on the Lee system until the 1860s, when William Cotton, also a Briton, devised a powered knitting machine able to put shape into the fabric it was forming.

Factory knitwear was first concentrated upon sporting uses. In 1900, the *Tailor and Cutter* decried a knitted sweater for cyclists as "neither smart nor sightly" and warned that any man found wearing one ran the risk of being taken for "a bounder". Advertisements about that time offered jerseys 'suitable for football and rowing' in stripes or plain. Such jerseys were long-sleeved with a roll collar.

It took the traumatic effects of World War I to liberate attitudes sufficiently for casual knitwear to gain full acceptance as proper accoutrement for the gentleman. Knitted waistcoats, often in canary yellow, were much in evidence in 1920. Some dashing fellows did away with the waistcoat altogether and sported beneath their jackets something new, the V-neck woolly pullover.

The prince of this new informality was the Prince of Wales himself. It was rumoured, even, that he was able to knit his own, though not surely the multicoloured Fair Isle pullover in Shetland wool with a jigsaw pattern that he later reflected was "the most showy of all my garments". He first wore it in 1922, at the Royal and Ancient Golf Club in St. Andrews, Scotland, and he was fond enough of it to have his portrait painted in it more than once.

What so pleased the Prince could not but please his subjects. Shetland wool pullovers in Fair Isle patterns became immensely popular, particularly among golfers, who wore them with plus-fours and a tweed cap. (Those straining to define a difference between 'pullover' and 'sweater' may be intrigued to learn that sweater is the older term, dating from 1882. Pullover did not appear in the Oxford English Dictionary until 1925, at the height of the Fair Isles fad.)

White or cream V-necks with club colours knitted into neck and hem were a standard accompaniment to sports jackets, blazers, or tweed lounge suits through the 1930s, and sleeveless, close-fitting slip-overs became established waistcoat substitutes for informal wear. As a signature image of the inter-war years, the diamond-plaid pattern known as argyle was applied to every description of knitwear, from sweaters to socks and even gloves.

Polo-neck and crew-neck sweaters, at first in heavy wools only, began to be seen in numbers from the late 1940s. A decade later came the bulking-up of sweaters and cardigans, worn much larger and looser than before. The plain polo-neck made its statement, often worn under a V-neck sweater or sports jacket to dispense with shirt, collar and tie. The knitted sports shirt, often half-sleeved, was another popular innovation, substituting for either regular shirt or sweater.

This post World War II period saw the development of knitwear on a grand scale. This response to an insatiable demand for leisure wear was made possible by the introduction of new man-made fibres and fabrics and new knitting machinery.

The 1960s have been called the decade of the knits. By its end, knitwear featured in every category of menswear, with the new machines creating knitted jackets, trousers, coats, and all manner of knitted accessory. Double-knit suits in polyester and wool or linen mixes made their début with the 1970s.

Traditional knitwear styles were enhanced by the flair of Italian designers such as the Missonis, who fully exploited the virtuosity of the new machinery. Subtle patterns in myriad colours delighted those who could afford them, much as the fancy Fair Isles had delighted the Prince.

STYLE

The emergence of sophisticated knitwear has brought a fluid new dimension to menswear. The sweater in its multiple forms is not only immensely practical and adaptable, it provides the gentleman with a legitimate opportunity to be adventurous.

The application of a dash of colour that is 'just right' can lend distinction to an otherwise safely neutral outfit, while obviating any sense of the regimentation which can come from being a little too 'correct'. However, such a personality-defining gesture can be one's undoing. Adventure implies risk.

Those gentlemen wishing to cut a dash must be prepared to experiment and to attend carefully to the opinion of others, rather than rely upon what they think they see in the mirror. Few men instinctively recognise what is best for themselves. Before (literally) pulling the wool over one's eyes, the following points need to be considered.

FIT

After substance, shape has to be carefully considered. Crew, polo, and turtle-necks obscure the prominent Adam's apple. They also conceal that wrinkly zone which besets most 40-somethings. A boat-neck expands puny shoulders. The Raglan-sleeved sweater, with seems that run from armpit to collar, has the contrary effect; it also gives an illusion of length to short arms and justifies shoulders that slope too much. Sweaters with some padding in the shoulders assist the pear-shaped person, but can render the broad-shouldered gentleman top-heavy.

Sweaters with horizontal stripes lend girth to the thin and minimise the height of the tall, but large gentlemen need to avoid them. Vertical stripes tend to elongate the body and thus have the opposite effects.

Quite the trickiest questions concern colour, with recent years seeing the rise of the professional 'colour counsellor' to assist those with more cash than confidence. Even the most conservative English gentleman, wary of anything bolder than navy blue, has surely by now become sensitive to opportunities afforded by the engulfing kaleidoscope of the modern world.

An important first step is to fight the strong male tendency to make block comparisons (the brown-goes-with-brown mentality) and to think instead in subtler terms of blending shades of a colour. Nothing is more personal to an individual than those colours which most flatter his person. While a gentleman may think vaguely of a match for the colour of his eyes, he needs to appreciate the profound effect that his skin and hair have in determining what will give him that special 'lift'.

This calls for experimentation and consultation. Try holding variously coloured garments across the shoulders and compare carefully the effects they have upon the face. Since many of us are colour blind to some degree, and many more are mentally blind to the realities of the mirrored prospect before us, this is the occasion to seek the opinion of a respected friend. The occasion, perhaps, to seek the opinion of a woman.

MATERIALS

The advantages of knitwear include generally fine wearing qualities, shape retention and an elasticity that makes for supreme comfort. Against this, they snag easily and are sensitive to heat, as all who have holed out to a flick of hot cigarette ash know to their cost. Holes defy repair, but a threaded needle pulled through a snag will draw it to the reverse side and tidy up the situation.

PURE NEW WOOL

Any wool sheared from a live sheep as distinct from being removed from a carcass or reprocessed from previous use.

LAMBSWOOL

Wool from lambs up to seven months old. The fibres are not only soft but have superior spinning properties.

GEELONG LAMBSWOOL

Wool from lambs up to five months old. Named after an Australian town.

SHETLAND

This homespun from the Scottish Shetland Islands is famous for its resilient, slightly coarse-textured knitwear.

CASHMERE

Leaving aside precious vicuna and rare alpaca, the best sweaters are made of cashmere, which is the wool of a goat. The very best cashmere was said to come from the beards of wild goats caught clambering over the Himalayan Mountains of Tibet, but China controls Tibet and China exacts prices that are steep even by cashmere standards.

Knitted cashmere provides warmth without weight, while imparting the softest of touches on skin and hand. A cashmere sweater can be knitted in 'single', which means a single strand of wool, to create the ideal flat texture upon which to work a cable or similar hummocky stitch. Cashmere dyes easily and well, though its lovely natural coffee-cream complexion means that it takes most sympathetically to off-whites, greys, and similar gentle shades.

It has been argued with good cause that those willing or able to afford just one luxury sweater would do well to pick a classic cable-stitched, four-ply cashmere in cream, with a V-neck. It 'goes' with just about anything.

Cashmere comes at a price greater than is apparent on the label. It demands gentle hand-washing, it does not long endure hard wear, and it has a nasty tendency to moult in ugly little pellets of fluff.

Pure, ordinary wool may fail the cashmere touch-test, but it is hardier and consequently more practical, and it can be spun as fine as cashmere. Lambswool shows off well in a colour cascade from bright and bold to pastel pale.

VICUNA

Best known as the most exotic of all overcoat materials, the extraordinary downy softness of the Vicuna fleece makes it particularly suitable for luxurious knitwear.

ALPACA

The long, smooth hair from this relative of the South American llama varies in colour from white to brown to black, of which white is the most prized. Combining extreme softness and lightness with strength and elasticity, it is knitted into precious shell-stitch sweaters.

ANGORA

The downy hair of the Angora rabbit has great thermal properties and makes lustrous, warm knitwear. The breed originated in France in the 18th century, but it is now raised primarily in China. The white, silky coat is sheared every three months to yield up to 500g of wool annually. The material is so delicate that it is difficult to process, so it is often mixed with merino wool to produce quality blends.

RAMIE

A fibre similar to flax obtained from a plant native to south-east Asia. It is often blended with wool or cotton to produce lightweight knitwear that feels cool even in hot weather.

BLENDS

Each of the wool types mentioned above is also available as quality blends, each offering its own advantages in durability and ease of care.

KNITTING TERMS

The difference between weaving and knitting is that in weaving two distinct threads of yarn, one vertical and known as the 'warp' and the other horizontal, known as the 'weft', pass over and under each other. Knitting has one thread which makes a continuous series of loops. Needles do the looping, drawing the yarn through a previously formed loop and forming fabric from the series of chain-like 'stitches'. In machine knitting, often at extremely high speeds, each stitch is made by a separate needle.

PLAIN KNIT
A stitch in which the yarn is pulled forward to form loops.

PURL KNIT
Anw inverse stitch in which the yarn is pulled from face of the fabric towards the back. The reverse of the plain knit stitch, producing horizontal rows.

PLAIN AND PURL
As implied, the first row is knitted plain, the second is purled, and so on. This achieves a smooth surface and is suitable for all classes of knitwear.

Yarn strength

Lambswool and cashmere are available in different strengths, one-ply to eight-ply. The greater the yarn strength, the higher the density and durability of the garment. One-ply yarns are exceptionally light and suitable for summer wear. Four to eight-ply knitwear is winter quality.

Intarsia

Inlaid design in which the pattern shows in solid colours on both sides of the fabric.

Jersey

Knitted fabric with slight cording on one side. It may be made of wool or any other fibre or fibre-blend. The term derives from the island of that name. Jersey is also a name commonly applied to tight woollen sweaters, which were first associated with the island's fishermen.

Fully-fashioned

A manufacturing process in which the number of stitches can be constantly varied in order to achieve a desired shape. This prevents bulging at the seams and also laddering.

SOCKS

HISTORY

Sock comes from *soccus*, Latin for a type of light shoe. Stocking comes from stock, a band of fabric; the wooden stocks that locked up medieval felons by their legs is another use of the term.

The familiar knitted sock is both a modern phenomenon and an ancient one, but it seems to have been lost in between, that being ever the way with socks. Socks knitted with a primitive cross-stitch have turned up in 2500-year-old Egyptian burials and in some Middle Eastern sites. Sometime in the 5th century knitting was introduced into Europe by the Arabs, but it did not loom large in hosiery until long afterwards.

Stock and sock, the long and the short of it, were for hundreds of years 'hose', or leg-piping – pieces of cloth or linen sewn together in the shape of the leg and either wrapped in place by binding, or hitched to an upper garment by laced ties, called 'points', which were pulled for a tight fit.

Then came the Renaissance and the dramatic developments of tailoring and fitted garments, which, in exposing the legs, brought hosiery into the light in bold and startling new ways. By the 1390s, hose were being joined at the top to form a primitive pair of tights, with a flapped pouch inserted at the crotch. This was the codpiece, cod being a term for 'bag'.

Chaucer was on hand to describe the provocative New Look through the eyes of his Canterbury pilgrims. The Squire had blue hose with leather soles and black hose to wear with his slippers; a parish clerk in the 'Miller's Tale' wore hose of scarlet; others had speckled legs, their hose in brightly contrasting colours. The Parson compared the effects of the frontal pouch to a bad case of hernia and the swell of buttocks to "the hind-parts of a she-ape in the full moon".

The codpiece, at times grossly stuffed and padded, remained in fashion for almost 200 years, until the Elizabethans finally cast it aside for 'trunk-hose' (a pair of baggy trunks) worn with, at long last, nicely knitted stockings. By 1589, clergyman William Lee had perfected his knitting frame, a machine to knit stockings that performed well enough to remain in use with few improvements for the next

250 years. The 16th century ended with gentlemen showing a full length of leg in knits in every colour imaginable.

Stockings were at their fanciest in the 17th century, drawn up to cover the lower edge of knee breeches and elaborately embroidered. Striped stockings were a feature of the 18th century, but then the veil descended with the advent of trousers in the 19th century. The sight of breeches and male calf encased in silk lingered in the twilight zone of Court dress, to be finally abandoned during the Second World War.

MATERIALS

Quality socks are usually made from dyed yarns, rather than piece-dyed later. Four-ply yarns are usual, the ply being the number of strands twisted together, with up to 16-ply in the case of certain materials.

SILK
There are silk stockings...and there are silk stockings. The determining factor is the intensity of the twisting in the thread. Apart from pure silks, inferior qualities and recycled products exist.

It is a fallacy that silk does not wear as well as other fabrics: it is the strongest of fibres, and stronger even than steel. Silk is an excellent non-conductor of heat, and if not quite as absorbent as cotton, frequent soapy washings in moderately warm water will keep it refreshed.

Wool
Only hard-wearing merino wool is suitable for socks. Other wool types are too soft and too fleecy for the task.

Cashmere
So soft and so warm, luxurious cashmere is unfortunately not hard-wearing, but with a strengthening of man-made fibre, it becomes much more durable.

Polyamide
Nylon socks which did not require darning were hailed as a boon in the 1950s and regarded with alarmed horror by manufacturers. Man-made fibres have steadily improved and diversified. A polyamide can be worked into the core of a natural yarn in such a way that it does not come into contact with the skin. A 20 per cent polyamide infusion can increase the life of a stocking fabric by four times.

COTTON

High-quality cotton socks are made from Egyptian Karnak cottons whose long fibre lengths (staple) permit the spinning of extremely fine yarn. The Egyptian variety was brought to the United States around 1900 and now thrives in the Caribbean region as Sea Island cotton.

The degree of warmth provided depends upon the closeness of the knit. A very fine stocking is warmer than a thicker stocking which is not so closely knitted.

Wool warms better than cotton. Cotton is more robust than wool. Woollen socks can be reinforced with cotton in an all-natural blend, though this cannot match synthetics when it comes to longevity.

STYLE

The more formal the occasion, the darker the stockings. In general, they should be darker than the trousers. A gentleman is always safe in black; never in white.

With evening dress, socks must be over-the-calf, black and they should be of silk, as is proper for the descendants of stockings worn with knee-breeches.

A Universal Dictionary published in 1744 recommended "sea-green, cherry brown, purple-red and umber" as appropriate for stockings, after counselling that the colour should harmonize closely with that of the garments being. Sea-green having been out of style for some time, we can dispense with this, but it is a fact that gentlemen of late have been dipping their toes into hues beyond the 'safe' range of black to dark blue. We are not, however, about to advocate the example of painter David Hockney's cheerful mismatches in two colliding colours.

For casual and less formal business activities, a pattern might please, but nothing vivid, please. Matching socks to tie can be effective, so long as the match is not too blatant.

The classic ribbed stocking is knitted on a four-plain, two-purl pattern, while certain elegant styles are knitted in purl stitch only. The basic rule is that the wider the rib, the more sporty the stocking.

FIT

Socks come in four lengths: short (15 cm), ankle (29 cm), calf (38 cm) and knee socks (more than 50 cm). There is an international standard for sock sizes, unlike the confusion attending shoe sizes.

For the right fit, calf-width as well as length of the foot has to be taken into account. A wide calf requires a larger-sized sock. It is also important to be aware that after a couple of washings, shocks shrink by half a size.

Short socks are for relaxing in, only. At all other times, the sock must be of sufficient height to maintain serenity between trouser and shoe. The danger is at its height when relaxing cross-legged: there must no risk of a glimpse of naked flesh.

MANUFACTURE

All stockings in the early years of the 20th century were manufactured with ribbed tops and held up with suspenders. Styles were conservative. Winter stockings were made of wool, and those for the rest of the year were of silk or lisle, a fine-quality cotton made from tightly-twisted, long staple yarn that has been given a sheen.

Patterned socks were rare until new machinery in the 1930s facilitated the knitting of one colour over another and the blending of colours. Elastic tops that did away with the need for suspenders also began to be a factor at this time, initially with socks that reached just below the knee.

Blends featuring man-made fibres as strengtheners for heel and toes were a big factor by the 1970s.

Socks are manufactured fully-fashioned in a 'tubular' all-in-one knitting process, from upper elasticated end to the top of the toe, which is left open to be finished by manual 'linking' in the case of quality hosiery. Also quite distinct from cheap 'uni-size' products, quality hosiery is manufactured on forming cylinders to various widths and lengths. They are then drawn damp over heated forms and individually inspected.

FAUX PAS
White socks for business
Exposed calves

SHOES

HISTORY

The first form of footwear was a wrapping of skins for comfort in the Ice Age. In hot countries, the sandal was devised thousands of years ago as protection against the burning sands. At some distant date the skin-bag was combined with the sandal to create the first true shoe.

Roman soldiers marched on an early form of hobnailed boot, with peek-a-boo toes. The neat solution of a laced slit was one of the lesser-known achievements of Byzantium.

The Crusades led to an exchange of ideas in footwear as in everything else, one result of which was the appearance in the West of the pointed toe, followed in the 12th century by the high heel. The first 'pair' of shoes, separately crafted to fit a right and a left foot, also dates from this period.

The pointy-toe craze persisted to ludicrous (60cm) extremes before an inevitable reaction rendered shoes squat, square and wider than at any time before or since. Heeled shoes made a comeback, welcomed by horsemen who could hook them into the stirrup, but even more by Louis XIV, who lacked height, if nothing else. Such was the Sun King's enthusiasm that the standard curved heel is still known as the French, or Louis, heel.

The 18th century reverberated to the thump of the cowhide jackboot (the 'jack' being a metal support), which was tamed by the dandies into civilised forms for the drawing rooms of Regency England. The early 19th-century gentleman was consequently shod in a most warlike manner. As well as plain top boots, he had a choice of high, tasselled Hessians, less decorative Hussar boots (also known as buskins), and Bluchers, which were half-boots with open laced fronts.

The Wellington boot, a far cry from the rubber 'Welly' of its destiny, was made of soft leather and designed to accommodate the new-fangled trousers. Buckles had been the major form of fastening until the adoption of trousers, when latchets (thongs) were used, though laces gained in popularity after the invention of the metal eyelet in 1823.

From the 1830s onwards, long boots were relegated

to sport, but the half-boot in various forms remained standard footwear throughout the 19th century, mere shoes not being deemed formal enough for polite society. As well as Bluchers, there were side-laced Alberts and front-laced Balmorals, named for the Prince Consort and the Scottish castle purchased by Queen Victoria in 1852. The Queen's love affair with Balmoral bore further fruit in the discovery of brogues, hefty highland footwear of untanned leather.

The invention of the sewing machine and the development of specialised machinery brought about the birth of the shoe industry about this time. Shoemakers were aghast. Gentlemen were unperturbed, and continued to have their footwear made by hand.

Low-cut laced shoes of recognisably modern style made their tentative debut as something for summer in the 1860s. A decade later, they were being worn with gaiters (spats) in wintertime by the young and audacious. They came in two styles, the Oxonian, otherwise known as the Oxford, and the Derby, but their acceptance in a strait-laced age was very gradual. It took the liberating effects of the First World War to put the shoe back on every foot.

Along with frock coats, boots were now the preserve of the very old and the incorrigibly conservative. In the brave new world of the lounge suit, Oxfords in plain or brogue became ubiquitous: so ubiquitous that the appearance in the 1930s of the Monk shoe was a welcome relief. The Monk style brought back the buckle after a long absence, while managing to match the basic Oxford for elegant simplicity.

Other departures were more radical. 'Reverse calf' (suede) was considered to be a sign of the cad, or worse, dangerously effeminate, until the Prince of Wales caused one of his sensations by wearing them to America in 1924. The Prince also favoured two-toned shoes (sometimes dubbed 'co-respondents'), another suspect style which became popular in the 1930s. Two-tones were to remain suspect, but by the 1950s suede was perfectly 'safe'.

The 'Peacock Revolution' and leisure explosion of the 1960s and beyond spawned a number of new styles, one of which bore the hallmarks of a classic in its matching of practicality, simplicity and elegance. The Moccasin, or Loafer, harked back to the primal origins of footwear while embodying the functional grace of true sophistication.

MATERIAL

BOX CALF

A robust black leather produced from the skins of calves (under 12 months) and used mainly for uppers. The best skins are reputed to come from beasts raised in the Alps. The same leather in brown is known as Willow Calf.

BUCKSKIN

Soft, pliable and durable leather of deer or elk with a distinctive grain.

CHROME LEATHER

Leather which has been tanned using salts of the metal chromium. A subsequent soap-and-oil treatment makes it very supple. Mainly used for uppers.

CORDOVAN

A rich, pliable leather made from the inner hide of the rump of a horse. It is tanned with vegetable substances and is non-porous. The name derives from Cordoba, Spain, which was famous for its leather in the early Middle Ages.

PATENT LEATHER

Cow, calf, kid or horsehide brought to a hard, lustrous finish by repeated applications of a thick lacquer, prolonged heat and rubbing with pumice.

SUEDE

The inner side of a tanned hide, buffed to give a fine nap effect. The name comes from the country first identified with it, Sweden.

FRENCH CALF

Waxed calf leather with a smooth, dull gloss. It is a feature of some quality shoes.

EXOTIC LEATHERS

The hide or skin of any animal, reptile, bird or fish can be turned into leather. Some remarkable leathers come from creatures as diverse as snakes and lizards, ostriches, crocodiles, sharks and carp, rhino and elephants.

STYLE

In order to be truly at ease and truly well-dressed, a gentleman needs to have his shoes made by hand. The process is long and ruinously expensive. To have a 'last' (the shoemaker's wooden model of the foot) made to the shape of one's own foot, and then to have that first pair of shoes or boots crafted to a state of bliss, can take between three to six months.

Custom-made shoes are a true investment. If treated with due respect and returned for re-soling when necessary, they literally last a lifetime. Natural leather after 20 years of wear and care attains a state of grace that mere words cannot describe.

This having been said, it is a fact that ready-made shoes have made great strides and there are establishments adept at making shoes that appear to be hand-made. The rule is, buy the best you can afford, or better still, cannot quite afford. There is no fate worse than to be found out wearing cheap shoes.

When it comes to choice of colour, the gentleman needs to be circumspect. The ancient Roman senators wore black shoes, and little has changed in 2,000 years. The classic spectrum reaches only from black to brown, with bordeaux, perhaps, on the outer limits. Black alone is proper for evening. Defy at your peril the maxim of the English gentleman: "Never wear brown after six."

Blue is acceptable, for leisure pursuits. Two-toned shoes (black and white; blue and white; brown and white) are strictly for the golf course or other sports place.

FORMAL SHOES

The formal shoe is required to be plain, black, and without a stitch of decoration, or perforation for that matter. It is made of fine polished calf or patent leather, and may be slip-on or laced.

The low-heeled, slip-on 'pump' with a flat bow dates so far back that the origin of the name has been lost. It was standard for grand receptions and balls when breeches were part of formal wear. Laced shoes were accepted after the First World War. Patent leather was preferred, but plain calf was increasingly seen from the 1960s.

OXFORD

The Oxford shoe is nowadays the classic companion of the business suit. Clean-lined, it comes in several sub-styles with historical associations. The 'bal', short for Balmoral, is a closed-throat shoe with laced front, and recalls the 19th-century boot of that name. The 'blucher' has an open-throat front, as did the boot named after the Prussian general who shared with Wellington the victory of Waterloo. The 'gillie' is a tongue-less Oxford, with lacing across the instep.

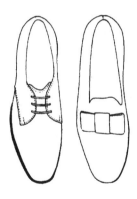

DERBY

This is basically an Oxford in reverse, inasmuch as the quarters and facings, which carry the lace eyelets, are stitched on top of the vamp, or upper. The seams are curved and the effect is more sporty.

WING-TIP

In contrast to the timeless, simple elegance of other classic styles, the Wing-tip is an exercise in intricate decoration. The name derives from the shape of the toe-cap, likened to the spread wings of a bird. This familiar style of the businessman originated with the elegantly curved toe-cap of a Victorian ladies' boot.

THE BROGUE

Tamed from its origins in the Scottish Highlands, the brogue is a Wing-tip Oxford with perforations on the tip and border seams. It traces it ancestry to a version of the Highland brogue introduced in about 1905.

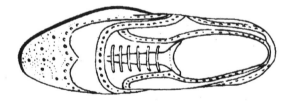

'Brogueing', or punching a pattern of tiny holes into the upper and double-stitching the seams, became a popular form of decoration, and brogues with fringed tongues were a favourite golf shoe in the 1920s.

Nowadays, a distinction is drawn between the Full-Brogue and the Half-Brogue. The Full-Brogue's perforation and decoratively-stitched seam runs right around, from toe-cap to heel. The seam of the Half-Brogue dips to the sole, leaving the back unperforated.

MONK

A charming legend has it that a 15th-century monk was first to create such a shoe with characteristic strap and buckle over the instep. In fact, buckled boots and shoes date from the 17th century, while it was not until the 1930s that the 'monk', or 'monk-front', style became popular as a welcome change from the Oxford.

MOCCASIN

This 'loafer', or 'slip-on', merits a place in any gentleman's wardrobe, always provided that it is made from quality leather by an able craftsman.

The name moccasin is of course associated with the North American Indian, whose soft and sturdy deerskins with designs distinctive to individual tribes had ritual as well as practical value. Curiously, we owe its modern popularity to quite another culture – that of the reindeer-herding Lapps of northern Scandinavia.

The story begins with Norwegian fishermen using their spare time to stitch together peasant shoes, some of which went on sale in London, where they were discovered by American tourists. There were two kinds, slip-ons called 'Weejuns' and a lace-up known as the 'Norwegian-front'. Americans had no doubts over what to call them and by the mid-1930s the moccasin manque was, according to *Men's Wear*, the "real man's shoe for a man's purpose in every conceivable situation and for every need".

The need reached upwards, so that by the 1960s a polished black moccasin was fully acceptable as a complement to the suit in every situation. Moccasins come in various styles, such as the Tassel Loafer and the fringe-flapped Kiltie. More useful if only because it is plainer is the Pennyloafer, whose little slit in the saddle is said to be the place to put one's 'last penny'.

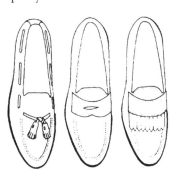

BOAT SHOE

Here is a good example of footwear evolution. With its water-repellent, oiled calf leather, rawhide lacing and non-slip soles for safety on slipper decks, the boat shoe was designed for the specific purpose made clear by its name. So much practicality coupled with a distinctive appearance and élite 'yachting' associations has made it a universal item of sporty footwear.

The deck shoe has also come ashore, for much the same reasons. It is made of tightly-woven air-permeable canvas and has soles like those of the boat shoe. It is useful for any leisure activity in warm weather. It may be worn with casual linen trousers or quality jeans.

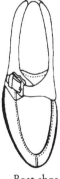

Boat shoe

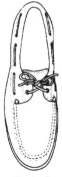

Deck shoe

MANUFACTURE

Between 200 and 240 separate operations go into the proper construction of a shoe made on the welt principle. By this we mean the careful stitching of leather upper to leather sole, as distinct from any of the grossly inferior glue or cementing processes.

Leather is the only material acceptable for footwear. In leather, nature gives us a material which ventilates our feet, just as it ventilated the animal it once protected. Perspiration, in the form of water vapour, rises naturally through innumerable tiny channels until it reaches the outside where it evaporates into the air.

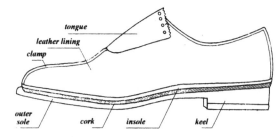

The outer leather sole is oak-tanned — a difficult, intensive tanning process which maximises resistance to wear and tear. Between the insole and the outer sole, there is a padding of cork, facilitating adaption in time to the contours of the foot. The best shoes are lined with high-quality peccary (wild pig's skin).

Through details such as these, the finest shoes are constructed in such a way that they become a virtual part of the anatomy of the foot, guaranteeing a very high degree of comfort and longevity.

QUALITY TAILORING
WELL WITHIN YOUR MEANS

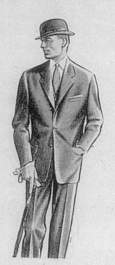

There's no greater name in Tailoring than Hawkes of Savile Row. Two centuries of skilled experience assure the true Savile Row style and quality. Men's requirements are met at most reasonable prices in Hawkes' Department for Immediate Wear. You cannot get better, quicker selective service—with the tradition behind it!

Hawkes of Savile Row

UMBRELLAS

HISTORY

As sword of the City, as tent, shield, lance and voucher of character, the gentleman's umbrella merits a respect denied the cheap and shoddy substitutes that have flooded the world's boutiques in recent decades.

The history of the umbrella is an exalted one. Over thousands of years, as its use spread through the Orient, it hob-nobbed with the high and mighty. The Golden Umbrella was the symbol of royalty in Burma, where the title of the ruler of Ava was Lord of the Twenty-Four Umbrellas. The Buddha rated one of seven tiers. In China, retinues of umbrella-bearers attended the progress of mandarins.

This clearly evolved out of the umbrella's relationship with the burning sun — even the word we use for it derives from the Latin *umbraculum*, meaning a shady place — and when it finally reached Europe late in the 16th century, it was as a sunshade. At that time the sword was the yardstick of the gentleman and it was only after the wearing of swords was discouraged that the umbrella made its début in the grasp of an English gentleman.

That gentleman was philanthropist Jonas Hanway, who in 1756 unfurled upon the streets of London a canopy of oiled cloth fastened over whalebone ribs. Hanway was ridiculed for his pains, and lambasted by the sedan-chair men, for whom rainshowers were a prime source of trade, but by the beginning of the 19th century the umbrella was an accepted part of polite society. We learn from Jane Austin that to be "equipped properly" for the resort town of Bath in 1818 entailed the acquisition of an umbrella.

The umbrella also caught the fancy of army officers, who took to using it to protect their splendid uniforms in bad weather. More remarkably, they also took to going into battle brandishing umbrellas in fetching shades of green and blue. Their commander, the Duke of Wellington, had himself inspected the troops from under a brolly, but this, he felt, was going too far.

The Iron Duke let it be known that he did "not approve of the use of umbrellas during the enemy's firing and will not allow gentlemen's sons to make themselves ridiculous in the eyes of the enemy". The officers nevertheless stuck with their umbrellas, off-duty anyhow, and an enduring tradition was born.

In 1830, the umbrella gained a royal connection when France's 'Citizen King' Louis Philippe exchanged his sword for a brolly in an unconvincing attempt to demonstrate democratic sensibilities, yet it remained a bulky, ungainly prop until the 1850s, when slim steel spokes were first applied. Now it could be rolled up tightly enough to simulate the highly fashionable cane, which had replaced the sword in formal wear.

From the 1880s, a rolled umbrella might be substituted for the cane in formal day dress, and no gentlemen of quality out for a Sunday stroll at the turn of the century would have cared to be seen without one or the other. It was usual, indeed, to have a wardrobe of canes – silver-topped black ebony for evening wear, malacca and rosewood for town wear, something more rustic for the country. Technically speaking, sticks made of ebony or white wood were 'walking sticks' while those of members of the bamboo family were 'canes', but any slender walking stick also qualified as a cane.

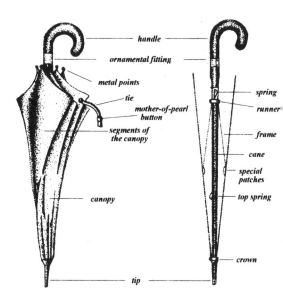

It was the advent of the motor car which caused the retirement of the cane, which by the 1930s was reduced to the role of accessory to top hat and tails. As the cane had replaced the sword, so now it was replaced by the umbrella.

Early in 1936, a newspaper photographer snapped Edward VIII near Buckingham Palace strolling under an open umbrella on a rainy afternoon. The picture was widely published, causing disquiet in Government circles. A furled umbrella was one thing; opening it, quite another. Some argued that a gentleman should keep his umbrella tightly furled at all times. At the sight of rain, it was pointed out, he could always use it to hail a cab.

Another ticklish point of umbrella etiquette concerned its use in the country, which was held by some to be appropriate only for gentlemen of the cloth. This debate shortly became academic, overtaken by the arrival from America of the big, boldly striped 'golf' umbrella, early specimens of which had been sighted there in 1937.

The march of science produced a tough nylon substitute for silk in the 1940s. This was followed in the late 1950s by the so-called Continental-style umbrella. A lightweight frame and cover enabled it to be rolled almost pencil-slim. The handle was of polished wood or stitched black leather.

The pop-up umbrella that sprang open at the touch of a button arrived with the 1960s. It was followed by the telescopic folding umbrella that slipped into a leather or plastic sheath small enough to fit into a pocket or briefcase; this so-called 'tote-type' umbrella was German in origin. The 1970s brought plastic bell-shapes and more shoddy oddities.

MATERIALS

Malacca, a soft and precious palm wood from the mountains of Sumatra, is used to make the handles of umbrellas fit for formal duty. It is repeatedly polished before being varnished. Beautiful, reddish Indonesian rosewood is an alternative choice. Whangee, a light and strong bamboo, ash, hazelnut, and cypress are among other materials used to make handles of distinction.

Swedish birch, being extremely flexible, is an ideal wood for the cane (shank). Maple, walnut, apple, chestnut, oak and cherry can all be used to fashion both handle and cane.

The frame is made of stainless steel, enamelled. Runners and plates are of bronze-plated brass. Silver or gold plate is used for the ornamental collar.

UMBRELLA SILK
This is a very closely woven nylon, which is especially water-resistant and hardy.

NATURAL SILK
A finished, water-resistant yarn is woven with four warp yarns and two weft yarns and rolled to create the watery appearance known as moire. The fabric

swells upon absorbing moisture to become extremely water-repellent.

STYLE

An umbrella is another of those ineffable expressions of character. It used to be said that robbers never carry umbrellas, and while this would be hard to vouch for any more (indeed, a poison-tipped umbrella was employed in a London street assassination not so long ago), the measure of dignity conferred upon one by a superior, hand-tooled umbrella cannot be over-estimated.

The choice of handle is most important. There are handles which have been mounted on successive frames, but better to purchase a truly superior umbrella in the first instance, and to have the frame recovered when necessary. Such an umbrella will last a lifetime and acquire a personality of its own.

The nature of the umbrella has prevented any drastic changes in style, though the handle has afforded opportunities for individualism. The curved, so-called 'crooked' handle has dominated down the years, while there have always been some gentlemen whose preference was for a handle set at right angles to the shaft, and some who have favoured a shorter handle with a knob. Rosewood, malacca, bamboo, silver and gold have led in handle-ware, with a menagerie of ducks', dogs' and horses' heads fashioned on quirkier examples. Ivory was once common, but, for understandable reasons, no more.

A natural handle is classic, though a metal shaft permits more slender rolling. The golden rule — the more formal the occasion, the darker the cloth — also applies to umbrellas. The black umbrella can be carried on business as on formal evening occasions. Brightly-coloured umbrellas are for sports and leisure pursuits.

Umbrellas come in several lengths. One must select that which one is most comfortable with. The handle needs to be comfortable to grip in an 'up' position.

Golf umbrellas are useful not only on the golf course. The shaft is usually of light metal. The handle may be curved or straight.

Travel umbrellas need not be of the grosser kind. There are superb designs, such as the malacca-wood and silver-banded 'Prince of Wales', which unscrew at the handle and tip for disassembly and easy transportation.

MANUFACTURE

The hand-made umbrella is a connoisseur's delight, its pedigree apparent to the discerning eye in dozens of subtle details. Sturdiness is of paramount importance, and all elements are manufactured and assembled with that in mind.

The handle is steamed and bent by hand, the process spread over several days to stabilise the form. Fitting shaft and handle together is craftsman's work of a high order, as are the insertion of the hand-filed runner and metal spokes, and the complex frame assembly. The eight segments of the canopy are cut and sewn by hand with yarn of high tensile strength. Securing canopy and frame is fastidious, exacting work.

A final touch are the ornamental fittings, usually of sterling silver or gilt brass and gold.

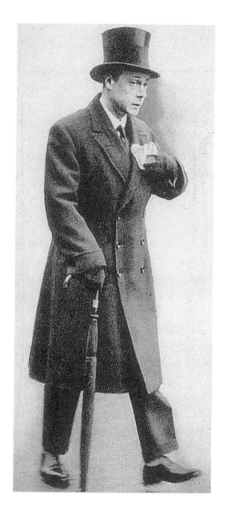

HATS

HISTORY

The hat is the most powerful item of clothing. It is
the tool of transformation, the weapon of authority, the badge of ceremony. No uniform is complete
without a hat, and this goes for the uniform of the
gentleman.

Despite this, the hat disappeared from most
wardrobes somewhere between the 1950s and
1960s, when it occurred to all manner of man that
there was something liberating and democratic
about going bare-headed. This was an extraordinary
turn of events, when one reflects upon the hat's
importance throughout history. In the 17th century, gentlemen even wore their hats indoors (including at meal times), and through the first half of the
20th century it was improper to go out without one.

The story of the hat begins as the story of felt. The
patron saint of hatters is St Clement, who put wool
in his sandals to relieve his blisters and discovered at
the end of his journey that the perspiration and

pressure from walking had turned the wool into a layer of felt.

The good saint notwithstanding, it is likely that early people discovered the felting process even before they learned how to spin or weave. Wool is still used, but the early hat industry was built upon a lighter, stronger felt made from beaver fur. This was bad news for the beaver, which was driven close to extinction in Europe by the time that North American supplies became available, only to become the cause of war between the French and English.

This brings us to the 18th century and the heyday of the three-cornered hat, now about to lose favour to a conical hat of country origin. Horsemen found the stiff round crown of the new hat provided some protection in the case of a fall, and as the crown was raised higher and higher, something about it appealed to gentlemen's sense of dignity.

We read in *The Times* how a Charing Cross hatter named John Heatherington appeared in the Strand on 15 January 1797 "in what he called a silk hat, a tall structure having a shiny lustre and calculated to frighten timid people". The spectacle drew such a crowd that ladies fainted, dogs barked, horses shied, and somebody broke an arm. Heatherington was fined 50 pounds for disturbing the peace. Enter the top hat.

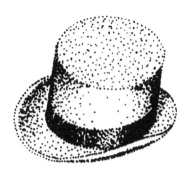

In the course of the next 50 years, the top hat became ubiquitous. Not only the gentry, but schoolmasters, policemen, train drivers, and sometimes even shepherds in smocks were wearing 'stove pipes' and 'chimney pots' by the mid-1800s.

In 1850, Norfolk landowner William Coke commissioned James Lock, the venerable London hatter, to devise something rugged for his gamekeepers, whose toppers kept getting knocked off when they were chasing poachers. Lock's adapted one of their own 18th-century riding hats and had the prototype made up by a Southwark feltmaker named Bowler.

The result was a snug-fitting crash helmet owing much to advances in felt-making machinery and to the conformateur, a French invention resembling an implement of torture, which when applied to a customer's head accurately recorded the dimensions. By the 1860s, this new kind of hat was widely fashionable as the 'bowler'.

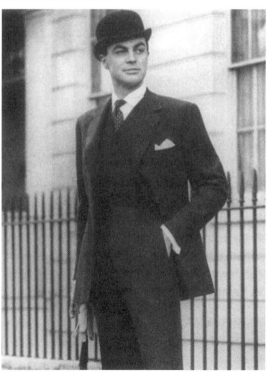

There were informal hats, too…the first deerstalkers and a velvet cap, the Glengarry, and romantic, dark felts with drooping brims, worn by the Pre-Raphaelities, revolutionaries, and Franz Liszt, who almost got himself arrested when he appeared in New York in one in 1851. Straw hats, first seen at the seaside in the 1850s, developed into the boater, a rage of the nineties. There were also exotic acquisitions from tropics: the Panama and the 'helmet' hat, based on the Indian sola topi.

The most significant development came about because an Alpine style briefly fashionable with women took the fancy of the future Edward VII during sojourns in Homburg, a south German spa. What became known as the homburg was a stiff felt hat with tapered, dented crown and a curved brim. The same shape in softer felt became the Trilby, named after a hat worn by Beerbohm Tree in the George du Maurier play of that name. The Fedorah, with roll-brimmed centre crease from front to back of a lower crown, was named after another play, staged in 1882.

The 20th century, dramatic in every other way, produced no new style of enduring popularity. Homburg, trilby and bowler were all worn with the new lounge suit, though not the top hat, which began its retreat to the rear of the wardrobe. In summer, boaters were worn with suits, or expensive panamas by those who could afford them.

For the 1920s onward, the hat trade's efforts were bound up in combating a growing tendency to go bare-headed. The solution was thought to lie in lightening the burden, and the result was a lighter, more resilient, easier-to-wear version of the trilby, known as the 'snap-brim'. Nattily turned down at the front and up at the back, the brim could be adjusted to personal taste. From the young Prince of Wales to the American gangster (who wore theirs with the brim effect much exaggerated), most men wore variations of this hat in the inter-war years.

The Prince also popularised a Tyrolean style in green with jaunty feather trim and a full-crown, almost floppy tweed cap that was in mocking contrast to the simple cloth cap that had become identified with working-class politics.

Following the Second World War, the hat industry clubbed together to promote the catchy slogan, "If you want to get ahead, get a hat", and launched a trimmed flat tweed cap and a trimmer trilby with narrowed brim and lower crown, but one no longer needed to wear a hat to look respectable, and fewer and fewer wore one for any reason at all.

STYLE

Mention Hollywood adventure hero Indiana Jones, and what immediately comes to mind? His brown hat, firmly affixed through thick and thin, from Lost Ark to Temple of Doom.

Now consider this: the Indiana Jones hat was built by Lock's, creator of the bowler hat and in business on the same fashionable London street for more than 300 years.

Such a remarkable conjunction bodes well for the long-term future of the hat, despite the momentary disregard it has suffered. Hats serve a practical purpose – a quarter of all body heat is lost through the head – and an important social one as an instrument of etiquette. For centuries, the hat was required to be doffed to a person of higher social status, or greater age, and always to a lady, and to her escort. 'Hat honour', it was called, and its niceties were quite as hard to master as the nuanced subtleties of the Japanese bow.

Instinctively, the gentleman craves a hat.

The hard-and-fast rule is that the less flexible the hat, the more formal it is. The softer the hat, the more casual is its appeal. The more formal, the darker the hat needs to be. In the aftermath of the Great War, when supplies of the hatter's plush needed to make black silk toppers were unavailable from Germany, those who determine such matters consequently put it about that the grey felt top hat, previously proper only for Ascot Week, would henceforth be correct wear for royal garden parties and society weddings, and so it has remained.

The opera hat is a collapsible silk top hat in matt black set in a spring frame. This accessory to the tail-coat is a descendent of the 'gibus' patented in 1840.

THE BOWLER

The bowler leads an active retirement as the symbol of an age now past. Books continue to be written about it, and it is the butt of limitless anecdotes.

Lock's persist to this day in calling it a 'Coke', after the customer who placed the first order. The French like to point out that it should by rights be called a Beaulieu, since that was the name of the feltmaker who built Lock's prototype, before he anglicised it to Bowler. In America, it is known as a derby, possibly after the 17th Earl of Derby, who wore it during his travels there.

Like the silk hat, the bowler suffered from the ravages of wartime shortage, of shellac in this case, but it managed to make something of a comeback in the 1950s, as part of regulation 'mufti' for Guards officers, for instance. Alas, it could not long escape the heavy burden of its storied past, including the slights of the likes of Charlie Chaplin, and George V, who never could stand the sight of one. Locked in a limbo all of its own, at once too highbrow and too lowbrow, it took a final gust from the democratising winds of change to sweep it from its last strongholds in the City.

Might one wear it still? Certainly. As a talking point, there is nothing quite like it, so long as one has the confidence to make the point.

THE TRILBY

This robust family of hats knocked the bowler off its perch in the 1930s, and can be spotted upon occasion demonstrating its practicality and diversity as it patiently awaits rediscovery.

Head of the family is the Homburg, elegant, stiff, in black or grey felt, with a turned-up and bound brim. Following the Second World War, it was increasingly seen with a dinner jacket. In the league of formality, it ranks after the top hat and bowler, but ahead of anything else.

The Anthony Eden is a tall-crowned black homburg, of softer material and great presence, made famous in the 1930s by the British Foreign Secretary. The Borsalino is the great Italian hatmaker's contribution to the trilby family, with characteristic triangle pinch to the crown.

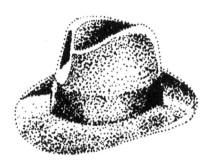

The pork pie, with low, round, dented crown, lacks serious intent, but goes with anything. The snap brim is a sporty, elegant trilby of soft, napped felt that can be shaped at will and is able to withstand being stuffed into a coat pocket.

THE BOATER

As with the bowler, the problem with the splendid old boater is that it is difficult to be taken seriously when wearing one, now that it has come to be associated with waiters in cheap 'theme' restaurants rather than with the Eton boating song. For the determined and the curious, it should be noted that the boater enjoys the privileged summertime right to be worn with dinner jacket as well as with sports wear.

THE PANAMA

This romantic reminder of Edwardian summers (when the king's panama cost 75 guineas, or several months of an average salary) merits a revival and may be on the brink of one, now that the dangers of sunburn are recognised. A quality panama hat is pleated from fibres of the jippi-jappa plant, a palm variety. The pleating is traditionally done under water in the cool hours of the day. A panama should be soft and silky to the touch – the best are reputed to come from Montechristi in Ecuador.

THE TWEED HAT

This sporty hat with narrow, floppy brim and soft crown that bends to one's desires was able to survive the hatless decades. It may be worn with casual suits or sports jackets.

THE CAP

In 1571, Parliament passed an act requiring all English males over the age of six (but excluding the nobility) to wear a woollen cap on Sundays and holidays. The law, intended to stimulate the wool trade, was repealed in 1597, but the cap with horizontal front brim of varying length has ever since been the leisure headgear, even if today it primarily sports the colours of American baseball teams.

FIT

Selecting the right hat may appear easy, since there is only one measurement to attend to. However, it is considerably more complicated than that. One needs to be aware, for instance, that under humid conditions a hat can shrink by up to one complete size.

The hat should settle into place without any need to exert pressure and there should be no hint of a wobble when the head is moved. In other words, one should hardly be aware of its presence.

	Centim.		English		USA		Points	
XS	52	53	$6^3/_8$	$6^1/_2$	$6^1/_2$	$6^5/_8$	$2^1/_2$	3
S	54	55	$6^5/_8$	$6^3/_4$	$6^3/_4$	$6^7/_8$	$3^1/_2$	4
M	56	57	$6^7/_8$	7	7	$7^1/_8$	$4^1/_2$	5
L	58	59	$7^1/_8$	$7^1/_4$	$7^1/_4$	$7^3/_8$	$5^1/_2$	6
XL	60	61	$7^3/_8$	$7^1/_2$	$7^1/_2$	$7^5/_8$	$6^1/_2$	7
XXL	62	63	$7^5/_8$	$7^3/_4$	$7^3/_4$	$7^7/_8$	$7^1/_2$	8

Achieving the perfect style match is a more exacting task, since it involves an interplay of vital statistics – the hat's brim and crown sizes juxtaposed with the wearer's height and skull dimensions. To cite an example, small men should beware wide-brimmed hats. The matter quickly becomes complex – pork pies, for instance, normally flatter small faces; Tyrolean hats need to be avoided by men with full faces – but theory can be no substitute for methodical trial and error.

MATERIALS

Hare and rabbit fur and merino wool are used to make hat felt. Some beaver fur is still used, though it has not been a significant factor since the depletion of American supplies in the first half of the 19th century.

MANUFACTURE

Making hat-felt was known once as the 'mystery', a dangerous process that destroyed the health of many of the skilled and proud journeymen who plied this ancient trade. The nitrate of mercury used to treat the animal hairs would raddle their brains, while the dust and fumes drove them to heavy drinking. 'Mad as a hatter' was a phrase with grim meaning.

Nowadays, steam is the agent of creation: lots of it, oozing from every vent in the factory. The hat's mysterious journey into existence begins in a dark and sour-smelling room filled with sacks and thick with slowly circling dust. The entire process from formless fluff to elegant fedora can take 10 to 12 days.

The raw ingredients are subject to dousing in vats, crushing, beating, rolling, steam-blasting onto whirling cones and compacting into damp, hardening felt blobs that are tossed and tormented, sunk in stiffening shellac, kneaded with steel hammers, moulded, pressed, ironed, drained of excess moisture and even sanded down in showers of felt dust.

Eventually, each embryo hat is given individual form and life upon a 'head' of wood, the hat-block press. After the mash of machinery comes the sleight of hand, patient and painstaking. Fingers of steams soften and give final shape to crown and brim, while deft hands guide the welt under a leaping needle and the hat is finished by trimming with band and lining.

UNDERWEAR

HISTORY

Like the continents that sink only to rise again from earth's heaving mantle, garments long submerged have a tendency to reappear centuries later, and the reverse is also true. It sometimes shows in a confusion of names.

Take the long, loose trousers worn by the barbarians of northern Europe and so mocked by the ancient Romans, who called them *bracae*. The bracae became 'braie', breeches, which over the course of time became shorter and disappeared under the Saxon tunic as knee-length linen drawers.

Many centuries later, the garment surfaced once more in the form of close-fitting pantaloons, which with the advent of wider trousers became shortened to 'pants', meaning tight underwear in English, though retained by Americans in its previous sense.

A similar story could be told of the word 'vest'.

The shirt is the supreme example. Up to the middle of the 19th century, it was always worn next to the skin and consequently it was essentially underwear. An instinctual awareness of this remains, in the sense of 'shirtsleeves' being a state of undress inappropriate for formal occasions. With the shirt removed from the tale, the story of underwear becomes exciting only in modern times, once Victorian industry and 20th-century enterprise and, finally, American imagination had been brought to bear upon functional unmentionables sometimes euphemistically termed 'small clothes'.

Bronze Age man sported a belted loin cloth, or so the limited evidence suggests, but from the time that clothes of recognisable form existed, the basic arrangement consisted of some form of simple linen tunic and loose linen drawers, closed by a string round the waist and often tied at the knees.

Needs of modesty aside, the purpose was purely sanitary: to protect outerwear from bodily secretion. With no dry cleaning, and less concern for personal hygiene, this was an important consideration. Though wool was sometimes worn next to the skin in northern Europe, the notion of underwear as a source of warmth is quite a new one. Until the development of closely-woven fabrics in the 19th century, one simply wrapped up with sufficient layers of extra outerwear in cold weather.

Linen was the universal choice, of poor as well as rich: the poor making do with coarser, thicker cloths, while the rich vied for the finest lawn or cambric or muslin, fine Holland cloth or Irish linen, sometimes so fine it was almost transparent.

Linen is strong, cool and absorbent. Silk was too expensive for all but the very rich, and wool is less comfortable next the skin and does not wash as well; it was believed that wool was more liable than linen to harbour lice. Cotton was not a major factor until its industrial development in the 19th century. The turning-point was the 1880s. For some time thereafter, the word linen was still synonymous with men's underwear.

Also in the 1880s, new industrial knitting systems began to release a flood of knitted underwear, much encouraged by health theorists like Gustav Jäger, who recommended its use at all times. 'Long johns' with long sleeves and legs enveloped the male form in the first decades of the 20th century, their wool weight depending upon the season, until common sense dictated their abandonment, in summer at least.

Cottons came to the fore, with more comfortably cut 'athletic underwear' offering from the 1920s a new approach to healthy practice. Elastic-banded underpants replaced tied 'drawers' and began to inch upwards, eventually to become briefs. In 1934, Clark Gable removed his shirt to reveal a bare torso in the Oscar-winning *It Happened One Night*, and men everywhere began to discard their vests in early acknowledgment of the power of Hollywood to determine popular style.

A form-fitting cotton 'training shirt' worn by U.S. troops in the Second World War became that post-war phenomenon, the T-shirt, worn at first as a vest and then as a sports top by young admirers of Hollywood idols James Dean and Marlon Brando. Underwear and outerwear had become one.

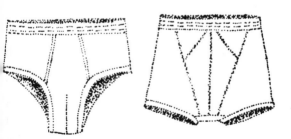

MATERIALS

LINEN

Linen is the material that touches the human psyche: our original raiment. The mummies of the Pharaohs of Egypt were wrapped in it; the priests of Isis and the Vestal Virgins wore it; it is the stuff of the Shroud of Turin. It was the stuff of gentlemen's underwear until supplanted by cheap and abundant cotton. It is cool to the skin, strong and absorbent.

COTTON

Cotton's pleasant wearing qualities, its easy-care characteristics, its durability, high absorbency, and above all its washability make it a natural material for undergarments. Long-staple so-called Egyptian quality cottons are best and are subject to various finishing techniques to achieve the desired feel and texture. Cottons used in quality underwear include:

FINE RIB a very fine knit of highly combed, linted and mercerised cotton.

DOUBLE RIB is extremely elastic, absorbent and kind to the skin.

SINGLE JERSEY a fine-spun cotton made into smooth-surfaced material that is light as a feather.

COTTON BLENDS

Gentlemen were intrigued in 1928 by word from America of a set of underwear which needed never to be removed: apparently one could stand in the shower and wash in it. The secret was revealed to be Rayon, known otherwise for a time as 'artificial silk', first of the man-made fibres. Rayon, incidentally, was coined from 'ray', to suggest a superior sheen, and the 'on' of cotton.

The 'Rayon Union Suit' of underwear thankfully proved to be a passing fancy, but by the 1950s gentlemen's loins were being used as test-beds for all manner of synthetics – nylon, largely, then polyester and cotton blends.

Adding five per cent of a synthetic with stretch characteristics, such as Lycra, improves the fit and shape-retention qualities of cotton, while a viscose blend will impart sheen and elasticity BUT underwear must breath, as nylon cannot.

SILK

'Silk is what you must wear if you want to reach God,' according to an old Chinese saying. This most luxurious of undergarment materials is light and cool. Silks with a small amount of twist to the threads – so-called radiums and tub silks – are used in underwear.

ANGORA

This is the wool most associated with thermal underwear, which keeps the wearer warm by trapping air between the threads. Highly recommended for skiers and those fearful of contracting rheumatism.

STYLE

There is a old saying that goes something like, "Show me your underwear and I will tell you who you are". An April 1935 edition of *Men's Wear* developed the theme considerably: "Underwear should have the presence of Apollo, the romance of Byron, the distinction of Lord Chesterfield and the ease, coolness and comfort of Mahatma Ghandi."

Behind this inspirational outburst was "sensational news of a new kind of garment" that had been reported in the American trade press in the previous year. These were knitted underpants of cotton devised by a firm named Coopers and modelled upon bathing trunks first seen on the French Riviera in 1932. Although with several inches of leg, it was audaciously form-fitting and it offered the 'gentle support' of a Y-shaped front panel. Here was something excitingly new, with "elastic fabric, no buttons, no bulk, no binding..."!

BRIEFS

Coopers became Jockey and by 1949 was advertising its patented 'Y-front' construction of knitted underwear as "scientifically perfected for correct masculine support". The loin-fitting shorts became waist briefs in the 1950s, and the needs of tight jeans allied with designer zeal advanced the cause with abbreviated hip-briefs, scanty sports-briefs, mini-briefs, scooped-out T-briefs and tinier still Tanga, not to mention 'posing pouches'. Sensible gentleman express their gratitude to America for the Y-front, and leave it at that.

BOXER SHORTS

The return to looser trousers has been accompanied by a welcome return of loose shorts, which even in the tightest of times never went out of favour with some gentlemen. The trunks of prize-fighters served as prototype for this type of underpants, which were another contribution of 1930s America to gentlemanly comfort. Boxer shorts should be generously cut and 'roomy' at the back, without a middle seam. They may be made of woven or knitted fabric.

VESTS

The compelling charms of Clark Gable's bare torso notwithstanding, vests retain a place in the wardrobe of a gentleman. Properly, a vest should be sleeved (short or long) and have a round neck. It should be cut longer at the back than the front and slightly higher at the sides.

SLEEVELESS VEST (SINGLET)

This style with comfortably cut-out armholes should also be longer at the back than the front. It may have a round neck or the so-called trapeze cut. It may be joined to the underpants and would have an absolutely smooth finish to the seams and flies, double-layered rear and front sections, finely bound edges to the leg sections and a band which will retain its elasticity throughout the life of the garment.

A quality vest has tightly finished seam-ends and smooth, flat binding.

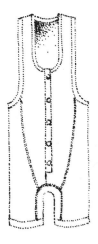

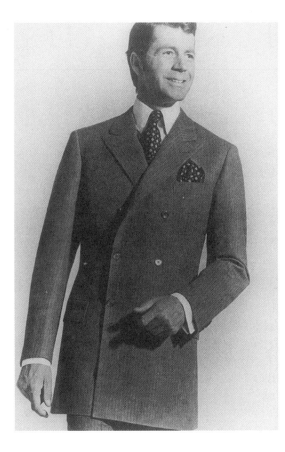

HANDKERCHIEFS

HISTORY

First evidence of the use of handkerchiefs comes from the appropriately named Chou dynasty in China. The fierce Assyrians, Biblical foes of the Israelites, were likewise gentlemen in this regard, while the Romans mopped their brows on sudaria, which translates roughly as 'sweaters'.

Nothing is known of the habits of the Britons until suddenly we come upon the courtiers of Richard II blowing their noses on their sleeves. The king urged an end to this practice, but was deposed.

The Italians, caught up in the clear new thinking of the Renaissance, were first to separate functions on the one-for-show, one-for-blow principle. The 'drapeselli' attended to business, while the 'fazzoletti' was purely for decoration. Fazzoletti might be carried in the hand, or tied to the upper arm, or even to the leg, pockets not yet being available.

In no time, fazzoletti were shot through with gold

and silver thread, trimmed with lace and laden with pearls. Ladies gave them to their lovers, mistresses received them from kings: the handkerchief as love-token was born. In some instances, sumptuary laws were enacted to try to control the excess. The town council of Halbertstadt in Germany decreed that "the handkerchief of the first estate shall not exceed two marks in value, that of the second estate not one mark, and the handkerchief of the third estate shall not be worth more than half a mark. Ladies and maidens using pearls to be fined one mark".

From the 16th century, the handkerchief of finest white linen found safe harbour up the sleeve, usually the left sleeve, of the gentleman of quality, while from the Americas came a new habit which greatly widened the use of handkerchiefs. This was snuff-taking, which began as a health fad, and became a mass habit until supplanted by cigarette-smoking in the 19th century.

A handkerchief for cleaning up and dusting off after partaking of a pinch of snuff was as essential an accessory as the snuff-box. Snuff handkerchiefs were dyed light brown or in bright colours to hide the stains, and the jaunty patterns turned out by the calico printers continued in fashion after snuff-taking had passed away.

The spread of cotton and advances in textiles meant that men of all classes could carry a handkerchief. As an instance, Jonas Hanway, umbrella pioneer and general fusspot, wanted "cheque handkerchiefs… however small" issued to every sailor in the British Navy as a sanitary precaution.

All that was left was to place the handkerchief on permanent display as the 'pocket handkerchief'. This came about as a natural consequence of jackets with breast pockets supplanting the frock coat.

With the 20th century, the handkerchief became what the menswear trade would call a significant style item, meaning that it was subject to a constant buffeting of fad and fancy. As Apparel Arts ominously put it: "The pocket handkerchief is an index of fashion change."

Officers returning from the First World War reverted for a while to placing the handkerchief up a sleeve, which is where they had been obliged to stow it when in buttoned-down uniform, but soon it was restored to the breast pocket, there to remain.

There was a vogue for fancy handkerchiefs in the 1920s. During the 1930s, a silk related in colour to the shirt and tie was frequently chosen. This tendency gave rise to a risible extreme, with handkerchief, tie, shirt, socks and even boxer shorts identically matched.

How to fold the handkerchief became an issue of lively debate. Some favoured the 'TV fold', a straight-line presentation identified with some television personalities, others the 'puff', or some arrangement of 'peaks'.

There were short-lived experiments, such as the 'speckerchief', an eyeglass case disguised as a furled pocket handkerchief. The 'Amore', promoted as "a distinctively new idea for every man of derring-do", was a singular achievement in bad taste. It consisted of a hand-rolled silk handkerchief bearing a pair of widely-spaced impressions to simulate lipstick smudges.

Such a handkerchief was of course never intended for smudging of any description. The one for blowing, of more serviceable construction, was tucked away elsewhere.

MATERIALS

COTTON
Most handkerchiefs are made of cotton. From sheer voile featherweights to spotted bandanas, there are plenty of beautiful styles from which to choose.

SILK
Silk looks splendid puff-folded in a breast pocket. It is less than perfect when called up for practical duties.

LINEN
The stalk fibres of the flax plant have a characteristic grainy texture. Fine 'lawn' linen is the traditional material for handkerchiefs.

HALF-LINEN
This is a cotton-linen mixture. It is both gentle and robust.

STYLE

A handkerchief may be called upon to perform many functions, but basically there are two, and these are contradictory. In seeking the ideal solution, one is tempted to invoke the *cri de coeur* of Beau Brummell: "Fine linen, country washing, and plenty of it."

Certainly, there are purists who hearken to a time when a crisp and generous square of white linen, simply folded, afforded every gentleman a full measure of style with a maximum of assurance, and no authority is comfortable with those who display a gorgeous plume of silk while secreting some base cloth (or wad of paper tissues!) for active duty.

Style is inconsistent with duplicity. It then descends to the vulgar. A handkerchief is not just an ornament. In the words of Hardy Amies: "It must look as if you use it; and you must."

The complexion of the handkerchief is another matter of some sensitivity. Some hold that it must be white, certainly with formal wear, though they will allow blue and pastel colours with business suits. Others are insistent that white is safe, but no more, and they advocate a bolder approach.

In necessarily contrasting with the jacket, the handkerchief is the final touch that completes the ensemble. It should not match the tie, but merely tone with it. It should likewise complement the shirt, or in the case of a striped shirt, the colour of the brighter stripe, but as in all such matters, one must beware impersonal adherence to fixed conventions. Style is in the end about flair, taste and feeling.

With this in mind, other colour clues to note concern borders, which on a white base draw attention to quality cloth; checks, which are a classic alternative amenable to lovers of white when dressing casually; decorative prints, the 'workman's cloth' of the 19th century, which offer unlimited scope for a dash of imagination on sporty occasions.

Whatever one's choice, the handkerchief must be of good quality and have a rolled hem. A monogram, the mark of ownership, is something of a status symbol, but it must be discreetly stitched and the handkerchief must never be folded in such a way that it shows.

VARIOUS FOLDING METHODS HAVE BEEN DEVISED. THEY INCLUDE:

THE SQUARE-END FOLD

The straight edge of the handkerchief parallels the rim of the pocket, revealing not more than 2 cm above the pocket. Handkerchiefs of all materials may be folded in this way. Most suitable for business occasions.

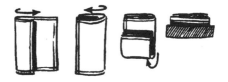

THE MULTI-POINT FOLD

It may have two, three or more points. The handkerchief is folded diagonally to the extent desired, avoiding too geometric a pattern. Most effective with linen or cotton.

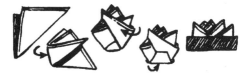

THE TRIANGLE FOLD

An elegant effect for formal wear can be achieved with all materials.

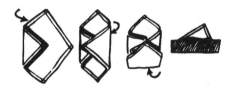

THE CRUSHED FOLD

The body of the handkerchief is puffed and inserted downwards to leave exposed a loose arrangement of points. Suitable for business as well as sporting occasion. Silk responds best to this arrangement.

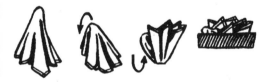

THE PUFFED FOLD

This is the crush in reverse, with the puff exposed with casual grace. Silk, again.

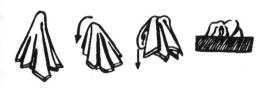

MANUFACTURE

Bales of raw cotton are washed, shaken out, combed, then spun and woven. The material is finished by singeing off loose fibres to produce a silky effect. Washing the bales in caustic soda (mercerising) makes the cotton lustrous and durable.

The cloth lengths are dyed and cut to size.

High-quality handkerchiefs are hand-rolled, i.e. the borders are turned and finished with fine stitches. The hand-stitched rolled border is the sign to look for. It is not to be confused with a machined border product.

LEATHER CLOTHING

HISTORY

The genus *homo sapiens* has been using animal skins as clothing for half a million years. This is adduced by dating flints used to scrape the flesh off the skins of animals that had been killed for food. It will be no surprise to students of the Bible, which records how Adam and Eve wore "coats of skins" in the Garden of Eden.

Since skins rot, primeval tailors would have to have been more or less constantly engaged in scraping until they could devise ways to preserve them. The simplest method was to stretch the skin out to dry in the sun until stiff and hard. By a stroke of genius, or more likely by accident, it was discovered that rubbing animal brains into the dried skin (and consequently treating it with a fatty oil) made it soft enough to wear.

The next monumental advance was to soak the skin

in tannin, tannic acid extracted from vegetable matter: in other words, to invent tanning. Tanning renders the skin immune to decay and shrinkage. The ancient Britons used oak bark for their tanning, and over the centuries very many other materials with special tanning properties were discovered; these ranged from chestnut wood to the bark of hemlock and mimosa.

In the Middle Ages, the Moors introduced tanning with minerals when they dressed goat and kid skins with alum and salt to produce a soft, bleached leather. Finally, by the 19th century, chrome-tanning was developed. This superior method employed salts of the metal chromium.

TANNING

The gentleman who takes a discreet pleasure in sensing that leather brings out the noble savage in him might be advised to hasten thorough this section, or skip it entirely. There is nothing 'natural' about the many industrial procedures required to put that soft, firm 'skin' on one's back.

Raw skins are first of all 'cured' by salting, then they are soaked, and the flesh and hair is removed. This process alone can take more than a month. Most skins are next treated with enzymes to render them soft and flexible and to smooth the surface. This is called 'bating'. The skins can now be tanned.

Chrome-tanning and vegetable-tanning are the two principal tanning processes, with innumerable variations of each.

Chrome-tanning is quick and creates the 'stretchability' required of gloves, clothing and shoe uppers. The skins are first soaked in an acid solution, then tumbled in a revolving drum filled with a solution of chromium-sulphate, or with a wide variety of other chemical compounds, each one able to impart a special characteristic.

Vegetable tanning is a slow process of weeks or months of pickling in vats; it results in firmer, more water-resistant leathers required for shoe soles, luggage, belts and the like. The two processes are often combined to produce leathers with a mix of advantages.

DYEING

After tanning, the leather 'stock' undergoes a variety of treatments according to its end use. Chrome-tanned leather for shoe uppers, for instance, is shaved to a desired thickness and then rolled in an emulsion of greasy oils. Vegetable-tanned leather for shoe soles is bleached, infused with a witch's brew of oils, Epsom salts, glucose and other substances, then lubricated with a hot, soapy emulsion and run through a rolling machine.

Dyeing is done in two principal ways. In high-quality aniline dyeing, the colours are allowed to seep deeply into the leather. In pigment dyeing, the leather is sprayed and a colour residue is retained on the surface to hide blemishes. A third alternative, semi-aniline dyeing, combines the two methods.

After dyeing, heavy leathers are coated with a finishing compound. Light leathers are sanded and buffed to remove surface imperfections. Buffing the reverse, flesh side raises the nap to create suede. To achieve a smooth surface, most light leather is waxed or treated with resins. Repeated coats of thick varnish give patent leather its high gloss.

Both of the basic forms of finished leather, 'grain'

and suede, can be made shower-proof.

The bulk of leather clothing in Britain has undergone a tanning procedure known as 'semi-chrome', which produces a firm finish. 'Full-chrome' leather is softer and sometimes known as 'Nappa'. Suede clothing may be semi-chrome or full-chrome.

STYLE

The niceties of so much technology, not to mention the significance of all the technical terms, are beyond the grasp of the layman, who must therefore trust in his instincts, and the certainty of his touch. Rest assured that a skin can be judged by its 'feel': the softer and more supple that feel, the better it is.

Most leather clothing is made from sheepskin, although many other skin types are also used. Cowhide is the least expensive. Lambskin can be costly, but rewards with its supple softness.

The gentleman, ever vigilant for errors of taste in other areas, must pay keenest attention when it comes to the consideration of leather wear. Leather is too louche a material to take risks with. It has no place in the formal wardrobe and yet it offers opportunities for casual elegance, indeed splendour, that should not to be denied. Just like a pair of bespoke shoes, a fine leather garment may be expected to gain in character with age.

Simplicity, both in cut and line, must be one's watchword. Avoid all flourish, fringe, or fussy detail. Cleave rather to a jacket of classic simplicity, straight draped to mid-hip, or to an equally simple blouson.

COWHIDE Cattle leather is very robust. It is used for shoes, belts and some outer clothing.

CAPE (CAPESKIN) Soft, fine-grain leather from haired (as distinct from woolly) sheep. The name derives from the original source in South Africa.

LAMBSKIN Leather from sheep is particularly pliable.

MOCHA Fine sueded sheepskin used primarily in glovemaking.

KID Soft leather made from goatskin. It can be tanned to a silky quality, wears well and is resistant to tearing. Much of it is made into suede. Kid leather produced from a young goat has a particularly close-textured grain and is thin enough for use as gloves.

ELK Scratches and scars are natural to this product of the wild.

PECCARY Also known as Hogskin. Peccary is made from a South American wild boar. It is very soft, pliable and air-permeable. Characteristically it bears the thorn and battle-scars of its previous owner. Imitation peccary is made from sheep and other skins. It is embossed with little holes that fake the real thing.

BUCKSKIN A soft-napped deer leather used for coats and blousons. Its gentle texture makes this a 'cashmere' among leathers.

REINDEER CALF The leather of the Scandinavian reindeer calf is soft as a glove and light. In spite of its fineness (Only 0.6 to 0.7 mm thick) it has great tensile strength, which makes it suitable for outerwear of superior quality.

LEATHER GOODS This term is applied to plastics and other synthetic materials used as leather substitutes. They lack leather's unique combination of qualities, but have a large share of the market, particularly in shoe soles.

JEWELLERY

HISTORY

There are peoples who go naked, but none who go
unadorned. The need for self-decoration is more
basic, even, than the desire to go clothed. Jewellery
is the oldest form of art, predating cave-painting.

Most of the ornamental metal processes used today
were known to the ancient Egyptians, as were such
familiar items as the signet ring. Noble Romans
were wont upon occasion to wear a ring on every
finger. Barbarian chieftains clanked from their load
of studded belts, buckles and bangles that bore witness to their rank and dignity. Among the Celts,
gold torques and bangles of great beauty were worn.

By the Middle Ages, pearls and gems were being
embroidered into clothing. As the craft of cutting
and mounting developed, ever more opulent belts
and pendants were fashioned, culminating in the
ornamental chain of office, worn over the shoulders.

The demand from wealthy families was such that

designs for jewels by celebrated painters such as Hans Holbein the Younger and Albrecht Dürer were printed and circulated throughout Europe – surely the first 'designer wear'. Through the 16th century, gold chains distributed by monarchs to the loyal nobility were much like the gold watches of later times.

The concept of having a matched set of accessories, or parure, was well established by the 18th century. A high-born gentleman's parure would consist of buttons, shoe buckles, sword hilt and a chained insignia of some knightly order. It was rather like having one's personal regalia.

Up to this point, gentlemen had out-glittered the ladies, but things began to change rapidly and radically, until court ceremony was the only occasion left for male ostentation – and the draught felt by the French Revolution put a chill even upon that. By the 19th century, a man was reduced to his signet ring, cravat pin and watch, with a brooch, perhaps, and fancy studs and cuff links to leaven the sobriety of his evening wear. A curious and quite long-lasting phenomenon was 'mourning jewellery', rings and brooches, sometimes containing locks of hair, in remembrance of departed loved ones.

The progressive process of denying the gentleman

his baubles continued into the 20th century, until he was down to his cufflinks, and even these were deemed unessential in the egalitarian nihilism of the 1960s. A reaction, naturally, was in train. Starting with the 'Peacock Revolution' of the late 1960s, the young began to sport chunky bracelets and gold neck chains. Among the lower orders in particular, chains and earrings (and dare one mention the occasional nose ring?) were worn with aggressive delight.

STYLE

A hint, the slightest glint, but nothing that smacks of ostentation: such must be the maxim of the gentleman. Understatement is path to the distinction.

Wristwatch, cuff links, wedding band or a signet ring, perhaps, are all that a gentleman ordinarily displays, and each piece should be as discreetly simple as feasible. 'Old' gold is easier to carry off than anything that flashes newness. Surely this is why a wristwatch with tails remains an awkward anomaly.

The studs, waistcoat buttons and cuff links of evening dress should ideally match, though this is not essential. What is important is never to mix gold and silver.

Chunky bracelets, gold chains, earrings and the like
are not the accoutrement of a gentleman.

TIE PINS

The tie pin (stick pin) is a comparatively new accessory of the gentleman, inasmuch as it dates from
the 18th century, when the artistically-bound neck-
cloth became the fashion. A two-inch silver or gold
pin with an ornamental head was used to hold it in
place; it might be topped by a pearl or precious
stones, or a glass or enamelled or engraved head. As
the 19th century advanced, the pin heads became
ever more imaginative, with fox masks and other
sporting motifs very popular. In 1901, the German
Kaiser sported a mourning pin bearing the initials
of his grandmother, Queen Victoria.

The stick pin today does formal duty with the ascot
of morning dress, or it may be used with a standard
knotted tie, or as a lapel decoration.

TIE CLIPS

The tie clip that clamps tie to shirt in the manner of a paper clip was an Edwardian innovation revived in the 1950s, not particularly popular nowadays. There are clips of gold and silver or plain metal, or enamelled in club colours. They are not to be worn with formal dress.

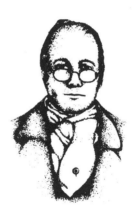

CUFFLINK

There is a French claim to having invented cufflinks, lodged on behalf of Louis IX in the 13th century. If correct, it was remarkably prescient, since there would be no need for them for another 600 years.

Even when flapping rectangles of soft white linen beckoned invitingly from the bottom of 19th-century coat sleeves, linked fasteners were uncommon until the 1840s, when they were not at first treated as an accessory in their own right, but as 'buttons'.

Only from the 1850s, with cuffs heavily starched and folded double in the style duly designated as the French cuff, did the 'golden twins' of Louis IX at long last gain recognition. The designs were English, however, not French.

This was in every sense the golden era of the cufflink. Yet not only gold, or silver, but pearls and gemstones gleamed with each flash of cuff, like shooting stars across the dark night of Victorian cloth. With the advent of the dinner jacket, less ostentatious sets of studs and links were worn, and as informality set in with the advance of the 20th century, the fancy cuff link retreated before the inexorable advance of the plain cuff and the humble button.

The classic cuff link consists of two studs linked by a chain. Studs joined by a bar instead of a chain are an alternative design. A single cuff-face, with plain clip to secure the unexposed inside cuff, is an American rationalisation.

Pearl, mother-of-pearl, gold, silver, semi-precious stones and intaglios are the stuff of ornamental cuff links. The antique trade is well-supplied with all sorts.

WATCHES

Watches have been worn since the 16th century, initially on a neck chain as a most luxurious piece of jewellery. The 18th-century gentleman carried his watch in his 'fob', a small pocket at the waistband of his breeches.

In the 19th century the watch was tucked into a waistcoat pocket and was such a symbol of the new age of commerce that a dandy might take pride in NOT carrying one. The gold watch attained its state of classic rectitude in 1849 with the introduction of the 'Albert', a watch-chain passed through a buttonhole and secured by a bar.

Wrist watches date from the start of the 20th century, but did not become common until the 1920s. The pocket watch remained the correct accompaniment for formal wear through the 1950s, and numbers were recovered from attics and antique shops and restored to active duty out of late-century nostalgia for old values.

The wrist watch has come to more than match the Victorian time-piece as serious body furniture. Cartier, Rolex and their like confer an instant identity upon those prepared to risk wrist-strain from the weight of precious metal involved in delivering their message.

Here again, the gentleman needs to take due care and not be swept into making a choice for the sake of ostentation alone. Select a design that is elegant enough to grace a dress shirt and yet does not jar with jeans: plain-faced, certainly, with Roman numerals, surely, and striking in its functional simplicity.

SPECTACLES

Anyone who considers it curious to include eyeglasses is either unaware or forgetful of times past, when the monocle was a most formidable social weapon. Even his greatest foe admitted of Victorian statesman Joseph Chamberlain, "he wore his (gold-rimmed) monocle like a gentleman".

The monocle was yet another casualty of the First World War, and eye wear went into sartorial eclipse until the 1980s, when 'designer frames' became the focus of attention.

Those whose business it is to know about such matters aver that girls most certainly do make passes at men who wear glasses; further, the style of frame that is most flattering to an individual's particular facial make-up can bring out character qualities not otherwise discernible.

There is a set of obvious structural guidelines. Horizontal frames, for instance, help to balance a long face; a vertically-aligned frame has the effect of stretching a round face. A high bridge lends stature to a short nose; a low bridge, set in the middle of the frame, 'shortens' a long nose. Rimless glasses are best for persons with small features. Wide, deep frames have been observed to make many a man look serious and sensitive.